Bioenergetics
of the Normal
and Malignant Cell

Bioenergetics of the Normal and Malignant Cell

By

Aurelian Udriștioiu

Cambridge
Scholars
Publishing

Bioenergetics of the Normal and Malignant Cell

By Aurelian Udriștioiu

This book first published 2023

Cambridge Scholars Publishing

Lady Stephenson Library, Newcastle upon Tyne, NE6 2PA, UK

British Library Cataloguing in Publication Data
A catalogue record for this book is available from the British Library

ISBN (10): 1-5275-9373-8
ISBN (13): 978-1-5275-9373-2

CONTENTS

PREFACE

The book Bioenergetics of the Normal and Malignant Cell is based on solid scientific information, gained through basic research in the country and abroad. Due to the wealth of modern data and because the system adopted in drafting the paper is very useful, especially practical in care physicians of all specialties, medical students, and staff working in clinical laboratories.

The theoretical and practical work is original content. The paper shows the great need for biological sciences in general and medicine in particular taking into account progress in pathophysiology. Appropriate authority, and novelty aspects treated, makes this volume constitute an important reference point for those studying and deepening problems of hematologic and metabolic aspects of the pathological body. The chapters convince the readers that these issues are addressed to medical personnel for all specialties, which can find the ideas on physiology and pathophysiology in the light of current concepts and modern principles.

In one chapter of the book, Bioenergetics of the malignant cell, is emphasized the energy levels of the metabolic pathways in malignant B and T lymphocytes and is presented the latest evidence from the literature, on cellular metabolites that may be oncogenic by modifying cell signals and blocking cellular differentiation. Advances in cancer metabolism research in the last decade have increased our understanding of aerobic glycolysis, anaerobic and other metabolic changes that are associated with cell growth and proliferation.

Blocking apoptosis in malignant diseases may be due to the high concentration of ATP from anaerobic metabolism. The energy difference between anaerobic ATP B and T lymphocytes in peripheral blood samples from hematopoietic malignancies measured by bioluminescence was 2.68 μM ATP, a value that appears as an energy transfer between normal B cells and T cells. The energy level can initiate the process of carcinogenesis by suppressing the activity of anti-oncogene proteins such as p-53 protein which is inhibited in its function of apoptosis and autophagy in the cellular anaerobic metabolism. It is concluded that anabolic metabolism in B and T cells in hematological malignancies are under complex regulatory control,

directed by receptors on the cell membrane, CD-5, CD-19, CD-20, CD-28, CD-38 and Zap protein Z, associated with an increase in signal transduction in cells transformed into malignancy.

The interests of doctors in all specialties, medical students, and staff working in clinical laboratories, from different countries on five continents, are based on the fact that this work is a large volume of data, experiences, and clinical and laboratory research. in a systematic and logical display. Due to the wealth of modern data and because the system adopted in drafting the Book is very useful, especially practical in care physicians of all specialties, medical students, and staff working in clinical laboratories.

Prof. Univ. Dr Viliam Lustig, MD, PhD, FCACB

CHAPTER I

INTRODUCTION TO CELLULAR BIOENERGETICS

The major energy source of the cell is the oxidation of the substrates of food principles in O_2 from the air, transported by the blood to the tissues. The living cell obtains its energy by oxidizing the hydrogen released from the organic substrate processed by the body, the formation of CO_2 appears as a secondary phenomenon, often dependent only indirectly on oxidation reactions, which ultimately lead to decarboxylation.

Numerous unknowns and many uncertainties over the years of medical research have made it almost impossible to delineate the preclinical phase of chronic disease from the initial state of health. The detection of biochemical changes in the body's apparatus and systems before their clinical expression has been quite uncertain through investigations conducted with the usual paraclinical means.

Modern methods of clinical and paraclinical investigation, by introducing new means of exploration, biological reagents, enzymes, coenzymes, antibodies, and antigens, try to solve the problems involved in basic research, with the following aspects: - the existence of persistent or transient disturbances in the molecular plane of the biological phenomenon that inevitably leads to the pathological alteration of the relationship between cellular structures and functions; - the precession of the biochemical and enzymatic phenomenon compared to the morphological one, such as the differentiation of the epiphenomena induced by the damaged structural support - oscillating states of cellular bioenergy in healthy and diseased cells. In the following, we will try to analyze these problems, while highlight, the bioenergetic complexity of metabolic processes in normal and malignant cells.

Most often, the energy is released in the form of heat released by the human body. In non-biological systems, caloric energy can be converted into mechanical or electrical energy. How biological systems are essentially

isothermal, it is not possible to use directly the heat released in biological reactions to carry out vital processes. Such processes as synthetic reactions, muscle contraction, and active transport, procure their energy by coupling with exergonic oxidative reactions. Processes that take place with energy release are called exergonic processes, and those that take place with energy consumption are called endergonic.

In living cells, the main macro-energic compound formed during exergonic reactions, which is used as an energy source in endergonic processes, is **ATP (or AMP-P-P).** Of great importance for specifying the direction of metabolic reactions and the energy exchange that accompanies them are the functions of the thermodynamic state: - **enthalpy (H)** or the total energy content of the system; free energy (G), which represents that part of the total energy of the system that can be completely converted into mechanical work in isothermal conditions and is the driving force of spontaneous reactions; - **entropy (S),** which is related to intrinsic characteristics (vibration, rotation, molecular translation) and which increases in all spontaneous processes, **[Figure 1].**

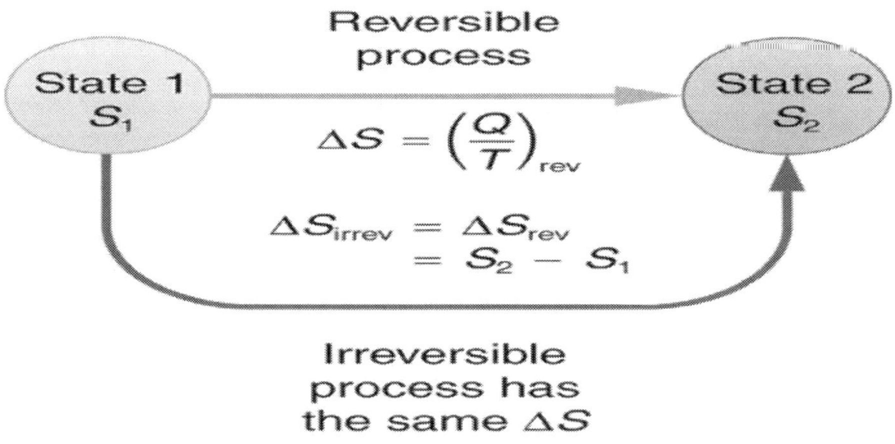

Figure 1. *There is an inverse relationship between free energy and entropy: when the entropy of the system increases, the free energy decreases.*

In the steady state, the entropy reaches its maximum value and the free energy the minimum value. free energy (G) is the part of the "usable" energy of a system and the entropy is the unusable (unavailable) energy, between these quantities there is the relation: $\Delta G = \Delta H - T\Delta S$ where T is the absolute

temperature K ° (273 ° C). ΔG will be higher the difference $\Delta H - T\Delta S$ if is the smaller ΔS and vice versa.

If the variation of the free energy of reaction A -> B has a negative sign ($\Delta G < 0$), meaning that the compound B has a lower free energy than A, the reaction is exergonic and therefore can take place spontaneously.

When $\Delta G = 0$ the system is in equilibrium, and the reaction proceeds without the release or consumption of energy.

The variation of free energy is influenced by the concentration of the components and therefore, in the case of equilibrium reactions it is a function of an equilibrium constant.

Consider the reaction A + B C + D; energy variation of the reaction will be: **ΔG = ΔGo + RT** log K where R is the general gas constant (1.987 kcal/mol/fence), and T is the absolute temperature. Going from the natural logarithms to the decimal ones we obtain: **ΔGo = - 2,303 RT log K.**

If more C and D are formed during the equilibrium reaction than A and B the equilibrium constant has a value and ΔGo is negative. In a reversible reaction, the compounds formed by the exergonic reaction are more than those resulting from the endergonic reaction. In a reversible reaction, compounds that are formed by the exergonic reaction generate energy that can be used to form energy-rich chemical bonds, which is the conservation of biological energy. Biosynthetic reactions are endogenous; for them to have, they must be coupled with exergonic reactions.

This coupling is most often performed by the synthesis during the exergonic reaction of a macro-ergic compound of the ATP type, which will take part in the endergonic reaction that provides the necessary energy. The energy contained in a chemical bond is equal to the energy released by the hydrolysis of that bond. According to the amount of energy released by hydrolysis, the chemical bonds can be divided into two groups: • energy-poor bonds, which release by hydrolysis below 5,000 horsepower; • energy-rich bonds highlighted by the Lipmann sign (~) which releases by hydrolysis over 5000 cal.

They play a key role in transforming energy by transferring it from one exergonic to an endergonic process. Among the macro-energic bonds, a privileged is occupied by the phosphate bond. This link is found in the nucleoside diphosphate and triphosphate through which ATP plays a central role (AMP ~ P ~ P). At the hydrolysis of a macro-energic phosphate bond

from ATP or ADP the standard free energy variation is ΔGo = -7.3 kcal/mol. The mixed anhydrous bond between phosphoric acid and an organic acid is also rich in energy. A standard free energy variation will be obtained by hydrolysis of the macro-energic bond. The phospho-enol bond is also very rich in energy.

For example, phospho-enol-pyruvic acid resulting from glycolysis releases a large amount of energy by hydrolysis (ΔGo = -14.8 kcal). The thioester bond, such as acyl-S ~ CoA, is another type of macro-energic bond. The guanidine-phosphate bond found in phosphocreatine is an important energy reserve in muscle. By its hydrolysis, ΔGo = -10.3 kcal is released. All these macro-energic bonds are of great importance, on the one hand, because they constitute a reserve of energy immediately usable by the cell, and on the other hand they make it possible to transform a radical together with the binding energy on another molecule. For example: ADP + P – enol-pyruvate ATP + pyruvate.

The frequency of this reaction increases in cellular neoplastic states when there is an intense degradation of nucleotides in the body with increased synthesis of IMP > AMP > ADP > ATP in the coupling, on the one hand, and on the other hand an intensification of anaerobic glycolysis with increased phospho-enol-pyruvic acid production. These metabolic pathways may explain the increased levels of ATP in the cancer cell, which is measured experimentally. In this way, the binding energy was conserved by transfer.

The continuous use of macro-energic bonds necessitates a mechanism for their permanent regeneration. This is achieved by coupling exergonic reactions in the cell, especially those in oxidative catabolism, with the endergonic synthesis of ATP in ADP + H3PO4. ATP in turn is used to provide the energy needed for endergonic biosynthetic reactions as well as to obtain the energy needed for any manifestation of cell life. Excess phosphate binding will regenerate ATP from ADP. When an organic substance burns "in vitro" the temperature reached is that at which C and H in the molecule combine directly with O2 in the air, according to the reaction:

CnH2m + O2 ------------> nCO2 + mH2O

The major energy source of the cell is the oxidation of the substrates of food principles in O2 from the air, transported by the blood to the tissues. The living cell obtains its energy by oxidizing Major energy source of the cell is

the oxidation of the substrates of food principles in O2 from the air, transported by the blood to the tissues. The living cell obtains its energy by oxidizing the hydrogen released from the organic substrate processed by the body, the formation of CO2 appears as a secondary phenomenon, often dependent only indirectly on oxidation reactions, which ultimately lead to decarboxylation.

Oxidation can be expressed in three different ways: O2 fixation, dehydrogenation, and electron loss. In the final analysis, oxidation is a loss of. electrons and a reduction of an electron gain. Any oxidation reaction (loss of electrons) simultaneously involves a reduction reaction (electron fixation).

Biological oxidations are always redox reactions in which H * or e- are transferred from one molecule (H + or e- donors) to another (H or e- acceptors). In redox reactions, the variation of free energy is proportional to the tendency of the reactants to donate or accept electrons. This is expressed numerically by the redox potential (or redox potential). A compound can only give up electrons to a compound that has a higher redox potential. This means that a compound can only be oxidized by a system with a higher redox potential.

The unevenness of the standard redox potential (ΔEo) is related to the variation of the standard free energy (ΔGo) by the reaction ΔGo = - nFΔEo, where n is the number of electrons exchanged in the redox reaction by a molecule, and F is the Faraday constant (96.399 kg or 23.06 kcal/volt). Because the value of the normal potential Eo varies with the concentration of H + ions and with the temperature.

In biochemistry, the Eo potential determined at Ph - 7.0 and T = 30 ° C is preferred. Cellular respiration is based on a remarkable enzymatic mechanism that allows the cell not to lose the resulting energy during respiration but to preserve it in a usable form stored in the phosphate-macro-energic bonds in ATP from where it can be easily transferred or released. The mitochondrial respiratory chain is a linear redox reaction sequence catalyzed by oxidoreductases in the inner membrane of the mitochondria.

Because cytochrome-oxidase located in the mitochondria is practically the only enzymatic system of cellular respiration in animals that reduces molecular oxygen, it turns out that mitochondria represent the energy centre of the cell. In aerobiosis, mitochondria generate almost all of the ATP used by the cell to meet energy requirements based on phosphorylating redox

processes. The force generated by this gradient is used to form ATP from ADP and Pi through a dehydration reaction involving Racker Coupling Factor (ATPase).

During cellular respiration, the passage of electrons through the respiratory chain determines the coupling of H + protons and their expulsion. In the contracted state of the mitochondria, the transporters in the respiratory chain are widely oxidized, the rate of ATP activation is high (ATP --> cAMP), the cation content is low and the protons are highly concentrated internally. In the swelling state, these parameters are reversals, the cations being accumulated inside and the protons released outside.

Ballooning can be prevented and contraction can be induced by the addition of electron transport inhibitors (oligomycin) or by oxidative phosphorylation decouplers. Oxidative phosphorylation in the respiratory chain is determined by the electrochemical potential created between the outer and inner faces of the mitochondrial membrane as a result of electronic transport in the respiratory chain. The process of decoupling oxidative phosphorylation isolates the production of energy from its preservation by preventing the formation of ATP from ADP + Pi

Most decoupled agents have some common physicochemical properties: they are fat-soluble substances that contain an acid group and an aromatic ring, and which seem to act by dissolving or discharging the macro-ergic intermediate or annihilating the cellular energy state by inhibiting electron transport (2, 4 dinitrophenols, cyanides, CO).

Inner membrane: NADH + H -> Fe S -> FMN -> b -> e -> a—> a3 -> 02: e-> 2H *> e-> 2H *> e

Mitochondrial membrane transport systems for ATP and ADP are inhibited by aromatic compounds (a cyclic aromatic compound with a free radical - O3SO in position 4 as well as by other antibiotics (free radical acid - OCH3^{+}).

In transport through the inner mitochondrial membrane, 6 C2% ions accumulate for the three phosphorylation sites along the respiratory chain, but the C2 + accumulation processes are not simultaneous but alternative. The development of the electronic transport process from NADH to O2 is carried out with maximum speed only when phosphate and ADP are present in the system in large quantities. By adding ADP, the 3rd state or active respiration, characterized by an increase in O2 consumption at the same time as the formation of ATP and ADP, is installed.

After the complete transformation of ADP into ATP, the speed of O2 consumption suddenly decreases, and the system returns to the 4th state. Stimulating O2 consumption is inhibited anaerobic glycolysis. The explanation for the phenomenon is as follows: Phosphofructokinase, an allosteric enzyme that catalyzes the regulatory reaction of fructose-6-phosphate to fructose-1-6-diphosphate, is inhibited by excess ATP as a final product of aerobic glycolysis and oxidative phosphorylation.

Decreased activity of this enzyme slows down the rate of the whole glycolytic process. In the increased production phase, ATP and other mitochondrial respiration products may function as inhibitors of anaerobic glycolysis. The main compounds, citrate and isocitrate, leave the mitochondria through transport mechanisms immediately through the tricarboxylic ring pathway (**Krebs**) and which, when they reach the cytoplasm, inhibit phosphofructokinase. In isolated mitochondria, volume oscillations, ionic motions, and oxidation-reduction states of hydrogen transporters can occur.

At the cellular level, we discover the chemical language of mutual information with important implications for fundamental biological processes such as multiplication, those based on excitability and contractility as well as heredity, mutagenesis, carcinogenesis or normal cell division. The energy stored in ATP is used in the biosynthesis processes of biomolecules with high specificity and a high level of organization. Their biosynthetic process takes place based on simple small molecule compounds, which come as such from the environment or catabolic processes. Of the four nucleic acid bases, adenine (A) has the highest resonance energy on the Π electron, followed by guanine. The basic nucleus of ATP is adenine, a nitrogenous base bound to a tri-phosphorylated ribose.

The important theoretical conclusion deduced from this situation is that the base resonance is higher for purine than for pyrimidine and that the highest value of the respective index has adenine. The π electrons appear to be responsible for the aromaticity of the ring hydrocarbon system. The double bonds of adenine correspond to the mobile electrons Π, delocalized, with orbitals asymmetric concerning the molecular plane.

The free energy of ATP is considerably higher than that released by the hydrolysis of low-energy phosphoric compounds such as glycerophosphates. The peculiarity of the macro-energic connection is explained by two essential factors: • the anhydrous character of the two macro-energic terminal links (pyrophosphates) of ATP and the properties of the products

that these bonds generate when hydrolyzed; in the anhydrous form, intramolecular electrostatic stresses are created which are released by hydrolysis.

The main factor that gives anhydrous bonds the macro-energic character is the resonant stabilization of acids resulting from hydrolysis. The multiplicity of resonant structures is an energetic stabilizing factor of the form. There are fewer resonant forms in pyrophosphate than in phosphate:

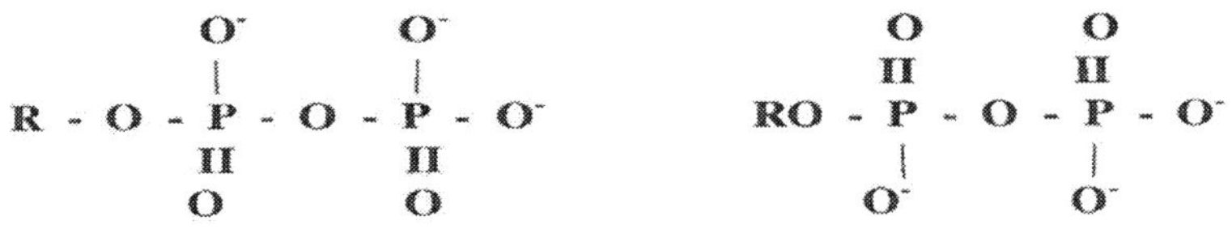

Resonance forms in pyrophosphate

Another structural feature that gives pyrophosphate its energetic character is the distribution of negative electronic charges (Π electrons in the pyro-phosphor axis) which is such that it generates electrostatic repulsions that are annihilated as a result of hydrolysis. Because both H3PO4 'and ADP3 anions resulting from the ATP + Pi ATP hydrolysis are negatively charged, they will be rejected so that they can no longer recombine to form ATP in the absence of an exergonic energy supplement.

The second category of macro-energic compounds of paramount importance for cellular bioenergy is, after ATP, phosphocreatine in muscle:

CPK PC + ADP C + ATP ΔGo = (-13 kcal / mol)

Other classes of macro-energic compounds with ΔGo of negative hydrolysis are phosphoenolpyruvate, thioesters (acetyl COA) etc. In all cases, the special electronic configuration in the macro-energic connection (or close to it), which will undergo hydrolysis is responsible for the strong negative value of the thermodynamic factor ΔGo.

Hormones are also factors in the mechanism of control and regulation of life cells, factors that belong to the extracellular coordinating systems superimposed on the primary intracellular ones. The binding of the hormone to the specific cellular receptor triggers the formation of an intracellular messenger molecule that triggers or depresses the biochemical activities characteristic of the target tissue:

Hormones known to work with cAMP in the two-messenger system are the anterior pituitary hormones: ACTH, LH, FSH, TSH, hypo-parathyroid hormone, and calcitonin. CAMP is a specific mediator in other types of cellular regulatory systems: - acts as a mediator in immune and inflammatory reactions; - stimulates the synthesis of antibodies, the phenomenon being proven in the regulation of the anamnestic response in vitro; - intervenes in the differentiation of B and T lymphocytes by cooperating with thyme-pectin and allergic hormones; - it also seems to participate in cell-mediated phenomena through sensitized T lymphocytes; - also participates in synaptic transmission in the nervous system.

In the regulation of cell division along with cAMP, cGMP also intervenes, both being involved in the regulation of gene expression during the cell cycle. They appear to act as inhibitors of the cell cycle phase by lowering the mitotic rate. In vitro, it has been shown that cAMP bacteria directly or indirectly intervene specifically on the operative site by removing the suppression of β-galactosidase synthesis.

The action of cAMP on nuclear transcription was shown to be mediated by a specific protein that can bind the nucleotide. This protein is called CRP (cAMP - receptor - protein). Models of the place-operon transcript have been released, involving cAMP, CRP protein and RNA polymerase. The functions of cAMP are influenced by calcium, which in some cases may increase the activity of the nucleotide and in other cases inhibit it. Very important for the regulation of cell life is the interaction between cAMP and other intermediate messengers of which prostaglandins have been recognized as first-rate regulatory agents. Prostaglandins, especially PGE1, serve as intermediate messengers between the surface hormone receptor and membrane-bound adenyl cyclase.

A general property of living matter is its ability to transfer energy to the needs of vital functions. In the phenomena of intracellular metabolic cooperation, it has been shown that a cellular biosynthesizing capacity can be transmitted by contact with a cell that does not possess this capacity. The hypothesis of free energy transfer without material carriers has also been issued within molecular structures.

All essential biomolecules that perform fundamental functions in living matter, proteins, nucleic acids, and macro-energic compounds, are composed of fully or partially conjugated (resonant) clinical systems, rich in delocalized π electrons (Pullman B, 1967).

One of the major features that electronic relocation imposes on compounds in which it exists is the increase of their stability, a state that defines the amount of resonant energy. These resonant molecules would produce, under the influence of radiation, stable states of excitation of relatively long duration. This reactive capacity was advantageous in the primordial conditions of life on earth by using solar energy with ionic discharges as the primary source for the synthesis of molecules, which led to biological molecules.

A free radical lipid peroxidation reaction (chemical species that have an unpaired electron in the outer orbital) can be propagated by phosphatide fatty acids in the mitochondrial membrane. Both the electronic transport in the mitochondrial respiratory chain (the phenomenon of ballooning - swelling) and the electronic transport through the OFMN system by the cytochrome P456 in the micro can be altered.

In membranes, however, the process of peroxidation can be stopped by vitamin E. Radical damage to the purine and pyrimidine bases can cause mutations and thus carcinogenesis. In the field of carcinogenesis, it has been observed that to be carcinogenic, a molecule must possess a K-reactive region (reactive aromatic bond) but be devoid of the L-para-reactive position region. These reactivities are expressed quantitatively in terms of the localization energy of the K and L regions, and some quantitative regions are established that allow the prediction of the carcinogenic properties of the substance.

Heidelberger (1973) indicated the formation of a strong chemical bond between proteins and carcinogens. Carcinogens are electrophilic reagents that establish covalent bonds with important biological macromolecules such as proteins and nucleic acids. Epoxides, which are highly reactive binding intermediates, are produced by microsomal hydroxylation of aromatic rings, which react as carcinogens.

Malignantly transformed cells continue to divide after confluence and reach a high saturation density. Malignant cell colonies then transfer the malignancy. In malignant metabolic pathways, pyrimidine, DNA, purine, hexose-monophosphate shunt, ribose-5-P generator, and key anabolic enzymes have increased activity, while catabolizing enzymes have increased low activity. In the anaerobic glycolysis sphere, the variation occurs inversely: the key anabolic enzymes have low activity while the activity of the catabolizing enzymes increases, thus ensuring a large amount of energy necessary for cell growth and division. In the normal cell it is

admitted that under various boundary conditions, the various parts of the glycolytic system are in a state of self-oscillation, which in turn can be a source of self-oscillation.

The focus of our study will be on the biosynthesis of ADP-ATP and its bioenergetic role. In all cells of the organism, the biosynthesis of ADP begins with the molecule ribose-5-phosphate, on which the skeleton of inosine acid (I.M.P.) will be built. In the first stage, R-5-P reacts with reserve ATP to form phospho-ribosyl / pyrophosphate (PRPP). The second participation of exogenous or endogenous reserve ATP occurs in the reaction between glycochol and PRA (B-5-ribosyl-1-adenine), forming GAR (glycyl amide nucleotide). The third participation of ATP takes place in the reaction:

FGAR (formyl – glycylamide - diribonucleotide) + glutamine + ATP --> FGAM + glutamic acid + ADP + H_3PO_4.

FGM + ATP -> AIR + ADP + H_3PO_4 FGAM contains in an open chain all 5 atoms of the purine imidazole ring. The next reaction has a cyclization reaction which will require the participation of an ATP molecule to form AUR (5 - amino-imidazole - ribose). In 4 carboxy - AIR the introduction of a nitrogen atom will also be done with ATP, consumption:

4 carboxyl AIR + aspartic acid + ATP ---> ISCAR + ADP + H_3PO_4

ISCAR - amino-imidazole-N-succinct-carboxy-amide-ribosyl. After the introduction of a CO_2-containing formyl group from the purine nucleus, the FAIR product is cyclized by removing a water molecule, resulting in the inosinic acid, the purine ribonucleotide, the primary product of intracellular biosynthesis. FAIR -> IMP + H_2O.

The biosynthesis of IMP and purine nucleotides is an initial endergonic process. 6 ATP were required for IMP biosynthesis if the process was initially started from rebozo-5-phosphate. Inosinic acid (IMP) is readily converted to adenyl acid AMP (by replacing the 6-position hydroxyl group of inosinic acid with an amino group derived from aspartic acid: IMP + aspartic acid + GTP -> adenyl-succinic acid, cleaved into fumaric acid and AMP. GMP is formed by the oxidation of IMP with the formation of xanthic acid and the consumption of 8 molecules of ATP.

The accumulation of purine nucleotides in the cell has the effect of inhibiting the biosynthesis process by a feedback mechanism. Aminotransferase is a multivalent regulatory enzyme and can be inhibited by ATP, ADP and AMP

by controlling the transfer of the amino group from glutamine to phospho-ribosyl-pyrophosphate. The biosynthesis of IMP and purine nucleotides is an initial endergonic process.

IMP biosynthesis required 6 ATP if the process was initially started from ribose - 5 - P. Ionic acid (IMP) is readily converted to adenyl acid AKP (by replacing the 6th position hydroxyl group of inosinic acid with an amino group derived from aspartic acid). IMP + aspartic acid -> adenyl-succinic acid -> cleavage -> = fumaric acid + AMP The accumulation of purine nucleotides in the cell has the effect of inhibiting, through a feedback mechanism, the process of biosynthesis. Aminotransferase is a multivalent regulatory enzyme and can be inhibited by ATP, ADP and AMP, controlling the transfer of the amino group from glutamine to phospho-ribosyl-pyrophosphate.

The phosphorylation in the above reactions occurs with the partitioning of ATP, which in most cases is the direct product of oxidative tissue phosphorylation. Thus, phosphorylation reactions are catalyzed in the first stage by nucleoside monophosphokinase and in the second stage by nucleoside di-phospho-kinase.

In living organisms, there are sometimes free purine and pyrimidine bases, most often from the total hydrolysis of the corresponding mononucleotides. These bases can be catalyzed by the formation of appropriate excretion products, but they are often preserved in the body and transformed into nucleotides that enter the metabolic circuit. This preservation process is very high in malignant cells.

Summarizing the above, we conclude that the biosynthesis of nucleotides from endogenous or exogenous nitrogenous bases can be done directly or after their conversion to the corresponding nucleosides. Direct biosynthesis involves the condensation of nitrogenous bases assimilated or resulting from endogenous catabolism, with 5 - PRPP - 1 under the action of nucleoside synthetase. Nucleoside - synthetases that catalyze the condensation of adenine, guanine, hypoxanthine, nitric acid, and uracil have been identified:

Riboză - 5 - P ATP —> APP 5' - P - Ribozil 1 - Pi + adenină —> AMP

exogenous or endogenous reserve. Indirect biosynthesis of nucleotides from nitrogenous bases after conversion to nucleosides is as follows: nucleoside:

1) Nitrogen base (adenine + R - 1 - P nucleoside - 1 - P phosphorylase nucleoside

2) Nucleoside + ATP nucleoside - 5 - P + ADP kinase. The nucleoside-5-P thus obtained can be converted to bisphosphate nucleosides by monophosphate and di-phosphate-kinase in the presence of ATP. The nucleoside triphosphates thus obtained are the immediate precursors in the synthesis of nucleic acids.

3) Nucleoside - 5 - P + ATP Nucleoside diphosphate + ADP

4) Nucleoside diphosphate + ATP Nucleoside triphosphates + AD In the phosphokinase 2 reaction the equilibrium is strongly shifted in the direction of phosphoric ester formation. Reactions 3 and 4, representing a transformation process, are reversible under the influence of phosphokinases. ADP is also formed from the phosphorylation of GMP, UDP, UMP, and IDP, with the help of reserve ATP or of exogenous direct origin:

GMP + ATP; GDP + ADP; UDP + ATP; UTP + ADP; UMP + ATP; UDP + ADP; IDP + ATP; ITP + ADP

Nucleic acids from food suffer degradation through a series of reactions such as those in tissues, in this way, the body, along with the formation of syntheses for nucleotide reserves, retains considerable energy reserves.

In cancer biochemistry, research on chemical carcinogenesis, enzymes of fundamental metabolic pathways, in all cells and their regulatory mechanisms predominates today, pathogenic chemotherapy aimed at inhibiting key enzymes and fundamental metabolic pathways for the transformation of neoplasia into normal states (DNA synthesis and degradation, synthesis and degradation of purines and pyrimidines, anaerobic glycolysis, hexose-monophosphate shunt). We can also talk today about the pathology of free radicals involved in carcinogens, [1].

CHAPTER II

ATP, THE UNIVERSAL ENERGY RESERVOIR

The vegetation of the planet we live on does not create energy but only one transforms the one received from the Sun. Our lives depend on this property of the green planets. Thus, the energy consumed by humans and mammals during life comes from solar radiation. The process of photosynthesis that takes place in green living matter is a large-scale example of the transformation of energy into nature.

The general equation of photosynthesis has been written as a reaction between carbon dioxide and water. light energy **CO_2 + H_2O --> O_2 +** organic matter green plants. Solar energy comes from the fusion of four hydrogen nuclei with the formation of two helium nuclei. **H Hc + 2c- + hv (energy)** Since the frequency of the radiation υ is inversely proportional to the wavelength, it means that the photons in the light with the short wavelength it is much richer in energy than long-wavelength light photons.

The photons in blue light are richer in energy than photons in red light. Pigments, present in plant tissues, must absorb the energy of a photon at the characteristic wavelength and then use this energy in photochemical reactions. A pigment after absorbing a convenient amount of energy (light) immediately releases an electron. By releasing the electron, the pigment molecule enters a state of excitation and at a later stage, there is a possibility that the energy absorbed in the system (the pigment molecule) can perform a photochemical reaction. Photon energy can be expressed in volts (eV). The energy of one mole of orange light (650nm) carries 1.9 eV. j / mol, **eV =9,65 x 104.**

White light energy contains 11.33 eV. Ultraviolet radiation contains 3,100 eV. In the process of photosynthesis, plants use the energy of sunlight to transform two inorganic molecules, extremely stable and poor in energy, CO_2 and H_2O, into unstable organic molecules but rich in energy and molecular oxygen.

Most of the organic molecules formed in photosynthesis are carbohydrates, which will polymerize to form polysaccharides. Thus, the formation of

glucose from photosynthesis can be represented by the equation: enzymatic system:

6CO2 + 6H2O 6 (CH2O) + 6CO2 with accumulated energy being 626 Kcal / mol.

The incorporation of CO2 with the formation of phospho-glyceric acid (PGI) initially as a product of photosynthesis is independent of light. Glucose will be formed from two molecules of phospho-glyceric acid, following reactions whose chaining is opposite to glycolysis. The process is carried out with the help of NADPH2 and ATP, formed during the light phase. In this case, oxidation of NADPH2 and hydrolysis of ATP to ADP + Pi take place.

But not only carbohydrates are formed from AGP but also amino acids, organic acids, fatty acids and glycols. AGP also serves to regenerate ribulose-diphosphate (which has been used in the formation of AGP). Trioses (glycerol phosphorylated aldehyde and its phosphorylated de-hydroxy-acetone isomer) by condensation can give rise to various phosphorylated carbohydrates with C6 (fructose, glucose), C7 atoms and finally with C5 (ribose).

There are many analogies between chloroplast phosphorylation and oxidative phosphorylation observed in mitochondria where ATP synthesis is associated with electron transfer. The energy required for the flow of electrons from chloroplasts is ensured by the absorption of light radiation energy by assimilating pigments, concentrated in the two points of the electron transport chain P650 and P700 (P comes from the pigment and its number from the light wavelength which the molecule absorbs). Each absorbed photon will conduct one electron through the inner membrane of the chloroplast. The main result that leads to the flow of electrons is the phosphorylation of ADP with the formation of ATR.

A. Phosphorylation of ADP in the plant cells

Following various research (Mitchell P., 1967) phosphorylation reactions in the plant cell are performed using enzymes (ATPases) implanted in the cell membrane. It is now accepted that the synthesis of several ATP molecules is associated with three protons in ATPases. ATP can therefore use two forms of energy, one from the proton gradient and the other from differences in membrane potential. The enzymes involved in ATP synthesis are similar for mitochondria, chloroplasts and bacteria. These enzymes, in electron

microscopy, look like globular bodies like protuberances on the surface of membranes. In plant cell chloroplasts these enzyme systems have been termed CFi1 • CF2 complexes oriented in the opposite direction to similar formations of mitochondria, bacteria, namely protuberances on the outer surface of membranes.

Electron flux is directed through the CFj • CF2 complex, and ATP is formed in the space between the inner and outer membrane of the chloroplast. In chloroplast, the CF] - CF2 complex requires the presence of three protons for each molecule of ATP synthesized, as opposed to mitochondria, in which the enzyme complex uses only two protons. Being an electron current, the phosphorylation that takes place from CF1 to F2 is called cyclic phosphorylation, as opposed to the phosphorylation that occurs in the transport of electrons from CF2 to CF1, which is linear.

All the transformations that take place after the carbon chain is charged with energy and H + from ATP and NADPH2, formed during the light reactions, no longer require a significant effort of energy and continue in the dark. Since these transformations in the reductive cycles of photosynthesis can also occur in the absence of light, the anabolic phase is also known as the dark phase of photosynthesis.

In the primary stages of photosynthesis, electron transfer, NADP production and ATP synthesis, O2 release occurs at the level of chloroplast thylakoids and is based on the accumulated bioenergetic background. The most important components of thylakoids are assimilation pigments, chlorophylls, carotenoids and phycobilin. Chlorophyll is a proto-porphyrin that contains a tetrapyrrole ring that has a cyclic system of 9 conjugated double bonds. These together with the 4 nitrogen atoms bound to the Mg atom correspond to the approximately flat part of the chlorophyll molecule (form a - form c). The main carotenoids, yellow or orange, are present in all photosynthesizing cells. In the leaves, their color is normally masked by chlorophyll, but in autumn, when the chlorophyll disintegrates, becomes visible, **[Scheme 1].**

The main carotenoids are p-carotene and xanthophylls. Carotene (C40 H56) is a hydrocarbon whose chain is cycled at the ends. Xanthophylls are oxygenated derivatives of carotene (C40H56O2). Carotenoids are located in the lamellae of chloroplasts in the vicinity of chlorophylls. In the process of photosynthesis, the energy absorbed by the carotenoids can be transferred to chlorophyll "a", which thus passes into an excited state (b, c), the carotin returning to their unexcited ground state. The resulting phycobilin has a structure close to that of pigments that come from light degradation.

The energy absorbed by phycobilin is transferred to chlorophylls to stabilize photochemical processes, **[Scheme 1]**.

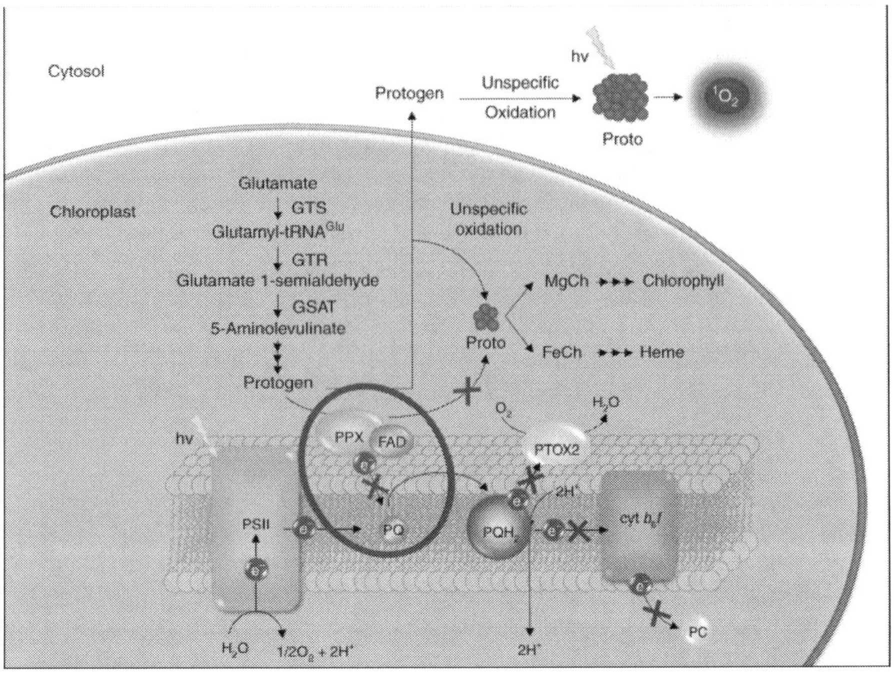

Scheme 1. *The scheme represents not only the natural balance of the process but also the energy balance. The atmosphere of the Sun is mainly made up of hydrogen.*

Photorespiration the process by which CO2 is released into the atmosphere has been considered a respiratory process of energy, however, it is suggested that this feature is not so pronounced because for every molecule of CO2 released into light 3 molecules of ATP-rich in energy are synthesized. Only 40% of the received energy is used in photosynthesis, 50% is the infrared region of the spectrum that cannot be absorbed by assimilating pigments, and the remaining 10% is lost through reflection, transmission and absorption.

Man depends solely on solar energy, used or current, to meet his growing energy and food needs. Solar energy is abundant, continuous, clean and free. That is why it is important to learn to use it most cost-effectively and effectively, imitating as much as possible the process of photosynthesis, which is carried out with extraordinary efficiency by plants, perfectly

adapted for photoconversion. As in animal cells, mitochondria in plant cells, due to the enzymatic equipment located in both membranes and matrices, play the following roles in cell biology: • partially ensures the degradation of synthetic cell glucose; • represents the headquarters of the Krebs cycle and of the respiratory chain that derives from this cycle; • are the site of syntheses and accumulations of substance.

There are two categories of ATPs in the plant cell: a) ATP of mitochondrial origin arising from oxidative phosphorylation; b) ATP of cytoplasmic origin that arises during anaerobic and partly aerobic glycolysis. Research (Niculescu et al., 1971) has shown that the mitochondrial membrane, which does not show a change in its intra-structural integrity, is much more permeable to bivalent ions (Ca2 +, St2 +, Mn2 +, Mg2 +) and less permeable to monovalent ions (K +, Na +). This permeability to cation anions leads to their accumulation in the matrix as well as on the inner mitochondrial membrane, a process materialized by a swelling of the mitochondria.

The movements performed by mitochondria by ballooning and contraction, depending on the nature of the ions in the environment and intramitochondrial, atmosphere, pH, changes in the cytoplasmic environment, etc. are in reality only movements related to the active transport of ions through the mitochondrial membrane. Studies have shown that the passage of mitochondrial membrane by cations and anions requires energy from either ATP in the extra-cyto-cytoplasmic environment or intermediate precursors of ATP synthesis, ex, DP + P2. One thing is certain: in the absence of light radiation, ATP is not initially produced from light:

LIGHT -> CHLOROPLASTS -> ADP + Pi -> ATP

Glucose biosynthesis also takes place with the help of light energy in the process of photosynthesis with the help of ADP synthesized from the three elements: adenine, ribose and phosphoric acid.

B. Biosynthesis of ATP in the human cells

From the histo-chemical point of view, the mitochondrial energy apparatus is represented by a set of intracellular formations of different shapes and sizes, with a double membrane (external and internal). The inner membrane is 1μ thick and has more intra-cytosolic septa, which increases their surface area, favoring surface catalysis. The essential function of mitochondria is related to the transport of hydrogen and electrons, oxidative phosphorylation and the Krebs cycle. In the mitochondria, there is an enzymatic assembly

called the respiratory chain that makes it possible to oxidize organic substances into the substrate, with the formation of water molecules. The substrate entering the respiratory chain undergoes the action of dehydrogenases, enzymes that carry hydrogen and trans-electron transporting enzymes. In the mitochondria, 300 enzymes have been isolated with a role in energy metabolism, among which are the enzymes of the aerobic catabolism cycle of energy principles (**Krebs**) as well as oxidative phosphorylation, **[Scheme 2]**.

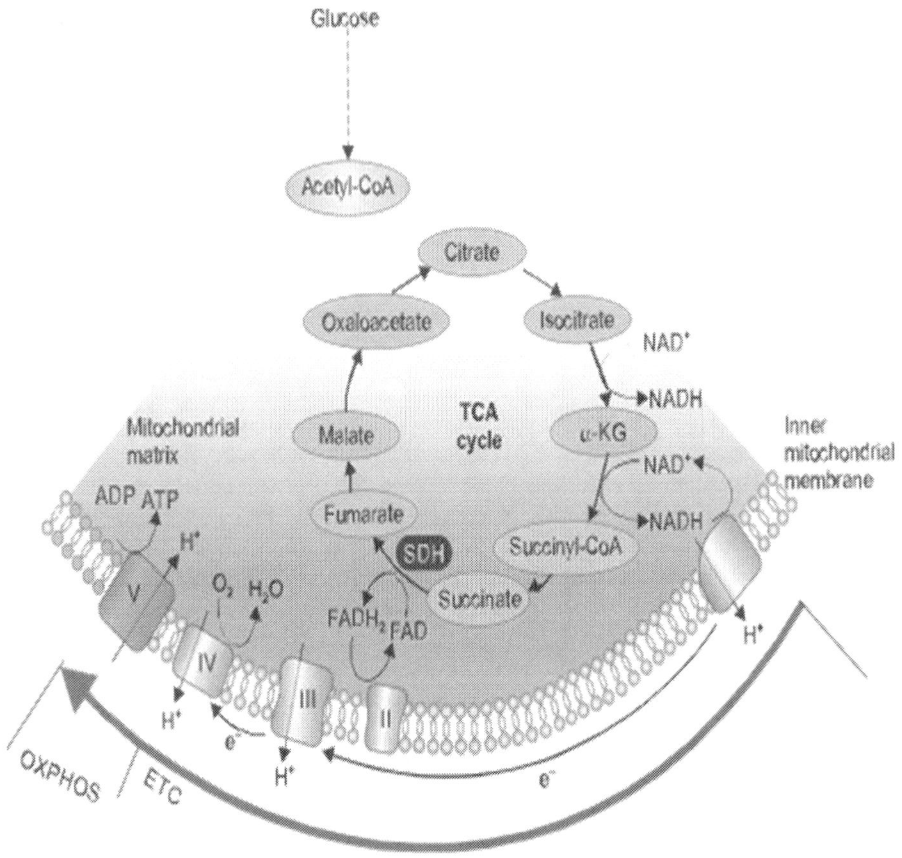

Scheme 2. *The oxidative process of water formation together with that of ATP formation is called oxidative phosphorylation.*

The reaction cycles release an energy of 52,000 cal/mol, of which almost 40% is used by the cell to synthesize ATP from ADP and inorganic

phosphate. ADP > ATP <. The highest amount of ATP is formed during carbohydrate metabolism coupled with oxidative phosphorylation.

The biochemical components of ADP are adenine, ribose, and orthophosphoric acid. a) Adenine is a 6-aminopurine formed on a purine nucleus. Adenine biosynthesis is performed either "de novo" from single metabolic fragments:

- CO_2, aspartic acid, glycochol;

- NH_3, glutamine; -formic acid, glycine, either from nitrogenous bases or nucleotides (ribose-coupled nitrogenous bases) from plant and animal nutrition as well as from nitrogenous bases resulting from the cellular catabolism of nucleic acids and nucleotides. Ribose is found in all cells with a nucleic acid composition and in the nucleotides of the animal and plant cytoplasm.

An important biological role is played by ribosomes as a component of nucleotides as enzymes. In these compounds, it is found in the form of furanone, glycosidic bound to apyrimidinic purine derivatives and phosphoric acid. Ribose, from a biochemical point of view, is a Penta-carbohydrate that can be absorbed from the diet at the intestinal level by simple fusion, an absorption process that does not involve an active energy-consuming mechanism. Ribose synthesis takes place in the human body via pentose-phosphates as well as in most green plants during the process of photosynthesis.

The pentose-phosphate pathway is the third major pathway for glucose degradation in the cells of the human body. The process begins with the oxidation of glucose-6-phosphate. Under the action of glucose-6-phosphate dehydrogenase (GPDH), 6 phospho-gluco-lactone is formed and then 6-phosphoglucose acid. In the next step, 6-phosphoglucose acid under the action of the enzyme 6-phosphogluconate dehydrogenase (PGDH) oxidizes and forms as final products CO_2, ribulose-5-phosphate and NAPDH> Ribulose-5-phosphate isomerase isomerized to ribose-5-phosphate

In some cases, the process can be stopped here from the oxidation of glucose-6-phosphate resulting in CO_2 and $NAPDH_2$, which enter the biosynthetic reactions that take place in the extramitochondrial cytoplasm and D-ribose-phosphate which is a precursor in mitochondrial synthesis. The global equation is as follows: G-6-P + NAPDBT ribose-5-phosphate + CO_2 + NADPH + 2H + In other cases, however, the resulting pentoses can be converted from hexoses into an independent sequence of reactions. The

pentose-phosphate pathway is not coupled to the respiratory chain and does not form ATP but is even consumed to activate glucose to glucose-6-phosphate. The different stages of this metabolic sequence have a role in the soluble phase of the cytoplasm and the products of the stages are implications in the biosynthesis of mononucleotides and nucleic acids, respectively. NADPH2 is the supplier of H2 and electrons in the biosynthesis of fatty acids, sterol compounds, etc. The penta-phosphate pathway is a strategic pathway used by the malignant cell for multiple, fast, energy-efficient cellular biosynthesis.

Ortofosphoric acid, H3PO

Phosphorus is the main biochemical element in its composition. In adults, the amount of phosphorus (P) required daily is 1.5 g and is provided by a normal diet. Phosphorus in the body is found in the form of various chemical combinations: -H3PO4 in the form of salts: Na, Ca, Mg; -compositions with pseudo-aldehyde function-monoesters of pentoses and hexoses; -organic esters and acids; -phospho-amino-lipid-type digesters; -pyrophosphoric acid derivatives:

Phosphorus absorption is in the form of soluble inorganic phosphate and occurs in the upper part of the small intestine. Phosphorus plays multiple roles in the body: - structural role in bone tissue, in the form of phospholipids that enter the structure of cell membranes; - functional role through its participation in the intermediate metabolisms of carbohydrates, lipids, and proteins; - energetic role through its participation in strong energetic bonds from macro-energetic compounds such as ATP, AMP, ADP phosphocreatine; - role of an enzymatic component of some enzymes NAD +, TPP, COA, pyridoxal phosphate. ATP formation occurs in the presence of specific enzyme systems, found in all living cells.

Given that many metabolic processes are not possible without the intervention of ADP and especially ATP, research has focused primarily on specifying the biochemical mechanisms that lead to the synthesis of these two groups of nucleotides. Thus, it has been established that in most cases ADP arises through a process of phosphorylation of AMP by ATP, a reaction catalyzed by AMP kinase:

AMP + ATP............ ADP + ADP
AMP-kinase

Regarding the biosynthesis of ATP, it was found that it requires precursors of ADP + Pi and can be achieved in aerobic as well as anaerobic cells. It has also been observed that to the same extent that ATP biosynthesis is performed, to the same extent there is a cleavage of ATP resulting from ATP + Pi with the activation of other intracellular chemical constituents as phosphate group acceptors. Living plant cells can synthesize ribose existing in the constitution of nucleic acids even in the absence of chlorophyll. Research on the biosynthesis of the purine and pyrimidine bases that make up the nucleic acids has shown that these bases are not found in the living cell as such, but only in the form of nucleotides (nitrogen base + ribose-phosphorylated).

In the "in vivo" synthesis of the purine nucleus it was stated that the carbon and nitrogen atoms of the nucleus have various origins: - N3 and Mg nitrogen atones from the glutamine amide group; - N1 nitrogen atom from aspartic acid; - N7 nitrogen atom from glycol; - C4 and C5 carbon atom resulting from glycol; - C2 and C8 carbon atom in formyl-tetra-hydrophobic (THFA); - C6 carbon atom from CO_2. Finally, the purine nucleus appears as a purine nucleotide, called inosinic acid or inosine-mono-phosphate (IMP). The starting point in this biosynthesis is the ribose-5-P, the support on which the basic components of the purine structure are fixed fragment by fragment. Throughout the reactions involved in this biological synthesis which suppresses 11 reactions, ribose-5-phosphate remains fixed on the final molecule which arises, i.e. on the inosinic acid. From inosinic acid (IMP), as a result of transmission reactions catalyzed by specific enzyme systems, AMP is born.

The synthesis of AMP requires GMP and GMP requires AMP, the excess of one component stimulates the formation of the other. AMP can also be formed during the synthesis of pyrimidine nucleotides, under the influence of the ATP synthesized from the components described above.

ATP+ Ribose-5-phosphate -> P-RPP + AMP

Also, starting from nucleoside-into-phosphate (DNMP), where d = deoxyribose, with ATP, AMP is formed. Transferases, d-NMP + ATP --> dNTP + AMP/. Biosynthesis of triphosphate d-nucleotides in eukaryotes occurs at the interphase, in the pre-syntactic period and the S-period, but before the depilation of the DNA molecule. Condensation of nucleotides into nucleic acids is not done from monophosphate molecules but from triphosphate nucleotides, an easy process in the cell because all monophosphate nucleotides, regardless of the nature of the nitrogenous

base, are converted easily in the nucleoside diphosphate and triphosphate by phosphate transfer from ATP.

GMP + ATP ------> GDP + ADP
GDP + ATP --- -> GTP + ADP

In the "in vivo" human body, the synthesis of AMP can be outlined as follows: 5 ATP Ribose-5-P ---> IMP ---> AMP ATP through the formation of carbamyl-phosphate from CO2 + NH3 also intervenes in the in vivo synthesis of pyrimidine nucleotides. Nucleic acids from food are degraded by a series of reactions similar to those in tissues. Pancreatic juice depolymerase converts nucleic acids from the cleavage of food nucleoproteins by the digestive enzymes of gastric, pancreatic and intestinal juice into oligo-nucleotides,

These are broken down by intestinal mucosal phospho-di-esterase into mononucleotides that will be hydrolyzed into nucleotides by intestinal phosphatase. Since the conversion of nucleotides to free nitrogenous bases involves phosphorylase, the reaction may occur intracellularly rather than digestively. Indeed, digestive juices contain an extremely small amount of free purine and pyrimidine bases.

Nucleotides and nucleosides (exogenous ATP, adenine-ribose) are transported in the blood to tissues that are degraded or used by the appropriate enzyme system in the synthesis of nucleic acids in the cells of those tissues or the synthesis of coenzymes. Urea, oxalic acid, formic acid, acetic acid, and propionic acid will form from the purine bases, each component taking a synthetic, energetic or excretory pathway. Adenine -> hypoxanthine -> xanthine -> uric acid -> excretion will form from the purine bases as well as from the unused energy from meat extract, and milk. Vegetables are poorer in purines, except for some vegetables, such as spinach and asparagus. Lipids and alcohol also indirectly cause the growth of purines and uric acid, respectively. We have shown above that the purine base is made up of very simple "Vivo" elements, namely glycochol (glycine), glutamine, aspartic acid, CO2, formic acid and ammonia. However, this assembly does not take place as a process but is done on the pentose-phosphoric skeleton.

Thus, at the end of the synthesis reactions, the respective endogenous purine will not take place, but directly a nucleotide, more precisely inosonic acid. Adenyl acid or AMP consists of ribose, adenine and phosphoric acid which is found in the form of three isomers: in tissues, AMP-5 and AMP-3.

Adenosine-5-phosphoric acid is found in muscle and is a physiologically active isomer. The enzymatic deamination of AMP-5 'gives inosonic acid consisting of ribose, hypo-xanthin (purine nitrogenous base) and phosphoric acid. Inosinic acid is the first nucleotide made up of muscle and is the precursor to other nucleotides in the body.

AMP can bind one or two molecules of phosphoric acid to form ADP and ATP, respectively. This phosphorylation process is an enzymatic process and occurs in the presence of nucleoside phosphokinases. As seen above, the second and third phosphate groups bind to the existing phosphate radical in the adenyl acid molecule through macro-energetic bonds. These bonds denoted by the symbol (~) have accumulated large potential energy reserves, which can be released by hydrolytic dissolution.

Thus, while the bonds stabilized by simple esterification reactions release 2-3 kcal mol of phosphate, the macro-energetic bonds can release by their hydrolytic release an amount of energy of 7.6-7.8 kcal mol of phosphate. Adenyl acids play a particularly important role in metabolic processes, as they can pass reversibly from one form to another by fixing or releasing a certain amount of energy. ATP ADP + H_3PO_4 + 8,000 cal. AMP is found in free form in the heart muscle, blood and brain. It is also an important component of enzymes with a special role in cellular oxidation processes.

It is well known that the role of the general energy reservoir in metabolic processes, is performed by ATP, which incorporates energy during the exergonic catabolic stages and provides it in the endergonic anabolic processes. It has also been pointed out that the absorption of DNA and RNA nucleic acids from food occurs predominantly in the form of mononucleotides and nucleosides. In tissues, nucleic acids can be similarly degraded to the nucleoside stage adenosine monophosphate. The richest food source is the viscera liver and kidney. Nucleosidases for purine nucleotides, which are cleaved phospho-group at the respective purine bases and pentose-1-phosphate, have been identified. Phosphorus, pentoses (ribose and deoxyribose), and adenine, resulting from the digestion of nucleic acids can be neutralized in biosynthetic processes.

However, the other purine and pyrimidine bases are degraded and eliminated. In intermediate metabolism, purine nucleotides, the major ones of which are AMP and GMP, are further hydrolyzed until the release of phosphoric acid, pentose and adenine or guanine, which are subsequently catabolized by specific mechanisms. In humans, the end product of purine catabolism is uric acid. AMP, under the action of an adenylate deaminase,

is converted to inosinic acid, IMP. Inosinic acid under the action of a phospho-mono-esterase is transformed into inosine and this under the action of a specific phospho-prylosis purine-nucleotide phosphorylase and in the presence of phosphoric acid releases hypoxanthine, also forming ribose-1-phosphate.

Hypoxanthine, under the action of the enzyme xanthine oxidase, is oxidized in the first stage to xanthine and then to uric acid which will be excreted from the body by the kidneys. Xanthine oxidase is an enzyme found in milk, liver, and intestinal mucosa. Structurally, it is a metal-flavoprotein containing FAD, molybdenum, and iron. In summarizing, can say that the viability of a cell, either in the plant or animal diet, can be stated intracellularly through the presence of ATP, [2].

CHAPTER III

THE ROLE OF THE ATP MG COMPLEX IN INTERMEDIATE METABOLISM

1. Role of the ATP-Mg complex in intermediate metabolism

In all living organisms, the immediate source of energy is the oxidation of glucose, in the bodies of higher animals and humans, glucose can be energy deposits in the form of liver or muscle glycogen. Along with glucose, as a result of the digestion of sugars in the small intestine, hexoses (galactose, fructose, mannose), as well as some pentoses also play the role of structural substances with specific functions. Absorption of hexoses in the intestinal mucosa is done by a chemically active mechanism after prior phosphorylation. In this biochemical process, the phosphate donor is ATP, and the reaction is catalyzed by hexokinase.

The highest synthesis of phosphorylation is galactose, followed in descending order by glucose and fructose. After phosphorylation, the phosphoric ester of the respective hexose (galactose, glucose, fructose) is hydrolyzed under the action of a phosphatase releasing the carbohydrate that passes into the bloodstream. The phosphorylation reaction is stimulated by adrenal cortical hormones, with adrenalectomy inhibiting these reactions. If in the body the degradation of carbohydrates starts from the stored glycogen, the biochemical process of cleavage of glucose molecules from glycogen is performed under the action of enzymes called phosphorylases.

Phosphorylase is present in tissues in two convertible forms: phosphorylase "a" and phosphorylase "b". Phosphorylase "b" is one of the enzymes in which allosteric properties have been found. The enzyme is active only in the presence of 5-cAMP which acts as an allosteric activator of enzymes, increasing its affinity for the substrate (glycogen and phosphate). CAMP arises from the action of cell membrane adenyl cyclase on cytoplasmic ATP. The reaction is stimulated by glucagon and epinephrine. Degradation of glycogen to glucose-1-phosphate is performed under the action of phosphorylase "a" --> phosphorylase "b".

Shifting the equilibrium to phosphorylase "a" accelerates glycogenolysis. This enzymatic conversion is performed under the action of a phosphorylase-kinase. Phosphorylase-kinase also exists in two interconvertible forms: - a very low-affinity form for phosphorylase "b"; - a form with increased affinity for phosphorylase "b". Phospho-ribulose-b-kinase activation is a dependent ATP process stimulated by 3-5-cAMP, the second messenger influencing various intracellular processes which in turn determine the physiological response of the target cell to the action of hormones: adrenaline, glucagon, ACTH, vasopressin, serotonin, (STH) and so on AMPc-3-5 can be hydrolyzed by a hormone-controlled phosphodiesterase, which gives the whole biochemical process a transient hormonal character. The conversion of "b" phosphorylase to "a" phosphorylase under the action of phospho-ribulose-b-kinase is accomplished by a process of ATP phosphorylation of serine residues in the "b" phosphorylase molecule.

Conversion of phosphorylase "b" to phosphorylase "a" appears to involve the simultaneous conversion of phosphorylase "b" dimer to phosphorylase tetramer "a" (containing four pyridoxal-phosphate residues per molecule) as phosphorylation occurs. The phosphorylase-b-kinase that activates the transformation is also activated by Ca ions, in the presence of a protein factor. The conversion of phosphorylase "a" to "b" depends on an enzyme called phosphorylase-phosphatase which is active by the phosphate radicals formed. Glucose-1-phosphate is produced by the action of phosphorylase "a" on glycogen.

The transformation of G-1-P into G-6-P is catalyzed by an enzyme called phosphoglucomutase assisted by a coenzyme, glucose-1,6-bisphosphate, a donor of a phosphate radical from the ATP molecule. phosphoglucomutase G-1-P ---> G-6-P ATP, Mg2 + The 1,6-bisphosphate glucose, which acts as a catabolic function in this reaction, results from a process of phosphorylation of G-1-P by ATP. G-1-P ---> G-1,6-P ß.

Following the transformations presented in the cells, glucose-6 phosphate accumulates in the glycolytic degradation sequence. When the degradation of the carbohydrate starts from the glucose monosaccharide, absorbed in the intestine and transported by the blood to the liver cells in the first stage, G-6-P is formed from glucose and ATP.

In tissue cells, exogenous or endogenous carbohydrates can undergo transformations that can be of two types: a) anabolic, in which the synthesis of carbohydrates from other compounds takes place, and b) catabolic In anaerobic degradation, a series of oxidation-reduction processes take place

in the cells of all living things in which energy is released, following processes by which they transfer hydrogen and electrons from the donor substrate to a hydrogen and electron acceptor, which functions as oxidant.

In anaerobic degradation, the final acceptor of hydrogen or electrons is an organic molecule, often formed during the degradation process. Glycolysis is therefore the process by which one molecule of glucose is transformed into two molecules of lactic acid. During glycolysis, the following occurs simultaneously:

a) the transformation of one molecule of glucose into two molecules of lactic acid;

b) a process of ATP formation due to the energy released in various stages of glucose transformation;

c) a continuous transfer of hydrogen and electrons through the intermediate transporters of H + and

d) which participate in these reactions; The transformation of glucose into lactic acid involves 11 catalyzed steps in the soluble phase of the cytoplasm. Within glycolysis, two stages can be distinguished:

a) Stage I - in which glucose is transformed into two molecules of triose phosphate (glyceraldehyde-3-P); this stage is the consumption of ATP.

b) Stage II - in which glyceraldehyde-3-P is converted to lactic acid, this process being coupled with the formation of ATP.

Without making a brief analysis of the **Embden-Meyerhof glycolytic pathway (E.M.P.),** we will further sublimate the stages in which ATP intervenes in the development of this process in the intact cell. The entry of exogenous or endogenous glucose from the blood tissue into the degradation glycolytic sequence requires its prior activation. This activation is done by phosphorylating glucose-6-P, under the action of ATP **[Scheme 3].**

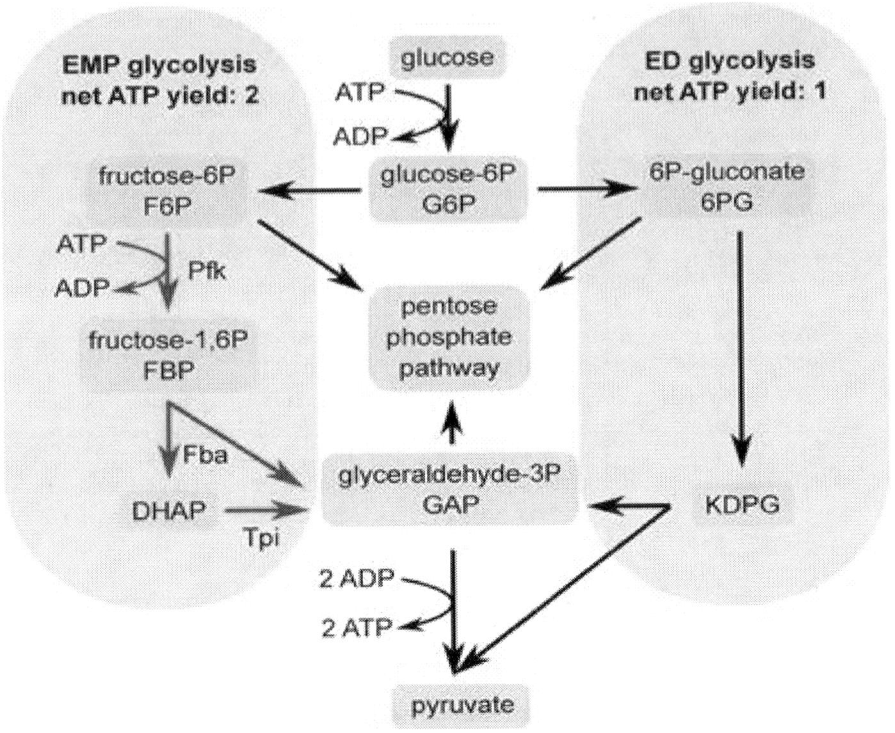

Scheme 3. *Embden-Meyerhof glycolytic pathway which it should be noted that there is relatively little free glucose in the cells, most of which is in phosphorylated forms in cycle Krebs,*

The reaction is catalyzed by two enzymes, hexokinase and glucokinase, and requires the presence of Mn2 + and Mg2 + ions, which form the corresponding salt with ATP. Of the two enzymes, the most active is hexokinase, which can catalyze phosphorylation and other hexoses: fructose, glucosamine, etc.

1. Glucokinase catalyzes only the phosphorylation of glucose, but with much lower activity than hexokinase. Due to the relatively large decrease in free energy in this reaction, the reaction is not practically reversible under normal intracellular conditions: hexokinase:

G + ATP --> G-6-P (ΔGo = - 4 kcal / mol) Mg2 + G-6-P

Hydrolysis will take place under the action of another enzyme, G-6-phosphatase. G-6-phosphatase:

G-6-P + H2O ---> G + P2 (ΔGo = - 3.3 kcal / mol).

The reaction is very important in the liver, as it provides glucose that will diffuse into the blood, being distributed throughout the rest of the body, in larger or smaller amounts depending on energy needs. 2) The next step of glycolysis is the isomerization of G-6-P into F-6-P (Δ Go = - 4 kcal/mol): phospho-glucose-isomerase; **G-6-P ---> F-6-P** ß.

The reaction takes place under the action of the enzyme phospho-glucose-isomerase, an enzyme which requires the presence of Mg2 + ions, which is perfectly reversible due to the small variations in free energy involved. 3) At a more advanced stage, F-6-P is phosphorylated to F-1,6 bisphosphate.

The phosphoryl residue is cloned by ATP, the reaction is catalyzed by phosphofructokinase and requires the presence of phosphofructokinase ions. Mg2 +, as the reactant is probably Mg-ATP.

FPK F-6-P + ATP --> F1,6-P + ADP (Δ Go = - 3.4 kcal / mol).

The reaction to form F1, 6-P takes place with a considerable decrease in free energy, which is why it is reversible under intracellular conditions. Phosphofructokinase is an allosteric enzyme with a regulatory role in the cell. It is stimulated by 3'-5 'cAMP and GMP and inhibited by excess ATP. Inhibition of the enzyme by excess ATP and its reactivity by cAMP is a direct link between the energy state of the cell and glycolysis.

Citrate, the substrate for the aerobic degradation of carbohydrates, is also an inhibitor of the enzyme. Thus, glycolysis intercalation is established - the Krebs cycle, which could be the very explanation for the inhibition of glycolysis by respiration. 4) The next step is the cleavage of fructose-1,6-bisphosphate with the formation of 3-P glycol-aldehyde and dihydroxyacetone phosphate. The reaction takes place under the catalytic action of an enzyme F - 1,6-bisphosphate aldolase) aldolase F 1.6 --> dihydroxyacetone phosphate + glyceraldehyde 3-P (Δ Go = 5.75 kcal/mol) The reaction takes place with energy absorption.

Aldolase, the enzyme that catalyzes this reaction is an HS enzyme, so an enzyme that contains hydrogen sulfide groups. These are essential for the activity of the enzyme. 5) Of the two triose phosphates formed, only 3-P glyceraldehyde, the phosphate can be subsequently converted to the

glycolysis reaction sequence. Dihydroxyacetone-P is previously isomerized, its transformation following isomerization. The reaction enzyme is tri-oz phosphate isomerase:

Isomerase dihydroxyacetone phosphate --> glyceraldehyde-3-P ß-- (Δ Go = 1.83 kcal / mol)

This reaction ends stage I of glycolysis. In the second stage of glycolysis, the degradation of glyceraldehyde 3-P to lactic acid takes place, during which ATP is formed. 6) This oxidation-reduction process is an essential stage of glycolysis, as in its course it takes place simultaneously with the oxidation process and a process of conservation of energy resulting from oxidation. It consists of the formation of a macro-energetic phosphorylated compound, namely 1,3 bi-phospho-glyceric acid.

Finally, the energy from 1,3 bi-phospho-glyceric acid is transferred to ATP, which is essential in biochemical energy. Oxidation of 3-P glyceraldehyde is catalyzed by the enzyme glyceraldehyde 3-P dehydrogenase (GAPDH-SH). This enzyme consists of identical subunits, each containing a HAD group. The active site of the enzyme contains an SH group through which the substrate is attached to form the enzyme-substrate complex.

The transfer of hydrogen and electrons to the NAD molecule then takes place. In this way, the aldehyde function is oxidized to the acid function corresponding to the thio-semi-acetal complex by an acid-enzyme thioester derivative. The resulting NADH2 and coupled with the enzyme is re-oxidized to a NAD molecule in the medium.

The acyl group is then transferred to an inorganic phosphate molecule from the intracellular medium, resulting in 1-3 bi-phospho-glyceric acid. The bound, re-oxidized coenzyme re-enters a new redox reaction.

The oxidation reaction of glyceraldehyde -3-P results in 1-3 bi-phospho-glyceric acid, a macro-energetic compound whose standard free energy of hydrolysis is higher than that of ATP, but cannot store it and give it up quickly. The global process can be written:

Δ Go = AG1 + AG2 = -43.05 + 49.32 = 6.27 kj / mol = 1.5 kcal / mol

It follows that the energy released in the redox process is conserved in the form of macro-energetic phosphate bonds from 1,3 bi-phospho-glyceric acid. Therefore, an exergonic process was coupled with an endergonic one. 7. Under the action of the enzyme pyruvate kinase, pyruvic phospho-enol

acid yields the phosphoryl group which is taken up by a molecule of ADP which is converted into ATP:

Pyruvic acid phospho-enol + ADP - > pyruvic acid + ATP (Δ Go = -7.5 kcal / mol)

The reaction is strongly exogenous. To exert its activity, the enzyme requires the presence of Mg2 + or Mn2 + ions as well as the presence of cations from aldehyde metals (K +, Ca2 +), but the physiological activator is potassium. The last stage of glycolysis is the reduction of lactic pyruvic acid under the action of lactate dehydrogenase (LDH) which has as coenzyme NADH2. The hydrogen and electrons involved in the reduction reaction come from the oxidation of glyceraldehyde -3-P. The reaction is as follows:

CH3 - C = O + NADH + H + -> H3C - CH - OH + NAD + COOH, (ΔGo = -6.0 kcal / mol).

Lactic acid is the end product of glycolysis and is formed in appreciable amounts in almost all organisms and organs whereas glucose degradation occurs in anaerobic amounts. Pyruvic acid, in the event of a local and temporary lack of oxygen or when the tissues have the necessary enzymatic equipment, is reduced to lactic acid.

Therefore, glycolysis takes place in tissues by creating a relative lack of O2 during the degradation of a molecule of glucose. 2 molecules of ATP participate, and 4 ATP are synthesized during the glycolytic process. Some tissues have an organic inability to rapidly degrade oxidative pyruvic acid.

Neoplastic tissues perform the so-called "glycolysis in aerobiosis", ex, a glycolysis in the presence of O2, but without its participation. The total energy balance of glycolysis amounts to -34.64 kcal/mol glucose (Total Δ Go = -34.64 kcal/mol). According to the free energy variations of the glycolysis reactions, during this process, there is a decrease of energy of 31.49 kcal/mol of glucose.

The molecule of glucose contains an amount of potential chemical energy in the amount of -686 kcal/mol. From these data, we can deduce that if during the glycolysis 4 moles of ATP are synthesized and 31.49 kcal are consumed, it means that 1 mole of ATP has a value of 7.87 kcal. Also, the remaining energy of 654.51 kcal will enter the aerobic respiratory **cycle Krebs** being dispersed in the two molecules of pyruvic acid. If glycolysis starts with glycogen to form F-1-6-bisphosphate, only one molecule of ATP

is consumed because the previous phosphorylation took place in the phosphorylase process due to the inorganic phosphate in the reaction medium.

2. The role of the ATP-Mg complex in aerobic carbohydrate metabolism

Pyruvic acid, formed in the terminal phase of glycolysis, is a nodal compound of intermediate metabolism. It can take various transformation pathways, depending on the conditions of the metabolic processes, linking the three partial metabolisms of the fundamental constituents of living matter (carbohydrates, lipids, proteins) and ensuring the specific dynamic balance necessary for any biological system.

a). Pyruvic acid can be hydrogenated under the action of lactate dehydrogenase due to hydrogen and electrons provided by NADH2, with the formation of lactic acid. It is the final stage of glycolysis, as seen above.

b). It can be decarboxylated simply under the action of thiamine-pyrophosphate, with the formation of acetaldehyde. This can be reduced under the action of NADH2 with the formation of ethyl alcohol. It is the process that underlies alcoholic fermentation, it can oxidize under the action of NAD, with the formation of acetic acid, as happens in acetic fermentation.

c). Pyruvic acid can decarboxylate under the action of an enzyme complex. The reaction results in Acetyl-Co-A entering the citrate cycle, **Krebs**.

d). Another mechanism of transformation of pyruvic acid is its carboxylation, under the biocatalytic action of biotin-enzyme, a process which results in oxal-acetic acid.

e). Pyruvic acid can be aminated and alanine will be synthesized, **£ *, (• / £ & /. ™ "• / 7.**

Acetic acid, In the presence of oxygen, the aerobic glucose molecule reaches CO2 and H2O through several stages. The final acceptor of hydrogen in the glucose molecule is atmospheric oxygen, even if it is directly involved in the process.

1). The transformation of glucose into pyruvic acid in the process of aerobic degradation W is analogous to the mechanism encountered in the glycolytic process, anaerobic. A peculiarity is that NADH2, formed in the oxidation

step of glyceraldehyde 3-P to 3-phosphoglyceric acid, enters the respiratory chain, generating three molecules of ATP, for each molecule of oxidized NAD.

2). Oxidative decarboxylation of pyruvic acid leading to the formation of acetyl CoA is a complicated process, catalyzed by a multienzyme complex, called the pyruvate dehydrogenase system, and occurs in the cytoplasm of the cell.

3). Oxidation of iso-citric acid is the next step in the cycle from which an oxalyl-succinic acid intermediate will be formed which is transformed into α ketoglutaric acid under the action of dehydrogenase and decarboxylase, respectively. isocitrate dehydrogenase:

Acid izocitric + NADP (NAD+) ---------> acid a cetoglutaric
ADP, Mg2+

An increase in the concentration of ADP in the cells, probably due to the consumption of ATP in endogenous reactions, stimulates the oxidation reaction of iso-citric acid and thus the speed of all the reactants in the cycle. This leads to a rate of hydrogen oxidation in the respiratory chain and the formation of increased amounts of ATP, respectively.

4). Oxidative decarboxylation of α ketoglutaric acid leads to the formation of succinyl-COA, the most important stage of the Krebs cycle, under the action of the α ketoglutarate oxidase system and several factors TPP, lipoic acid, CoA, NAD + or NADP +, ADP, GDP and H3PO4.

The macro-energetic thioester bond of succinyl CoA is converted to the macro-energetic phosphate bond by the formation of ATP, through a phosphorylation reaction at the substrate core. The energy contained in the macro-energetic thioester bond is thus stored in the macro-energetic phosphate bond in the ATP molecule. TPP A Ketoglutaric acid ---> succinyl Co-A. The energy in this reaction is Δ Go = - 8.0 kcal / mol:

Succinyl CoA + Pi + GDP ---> succinate + GTP + HS - CoA ß; Δ Go = - 7.0 kcal / mol GTP + ADP -> GDP + ATP

This formation of ATP, which is not associated with the respiratory chain - is called substrate phosphorylation.

5). Oxidation of succinic acid to fumaric acid takes place through the action of the succinate-oxidase complex and some factors: cytochromes, b, c, a3,

FAD: SUCCINATE Fumaric acid + FAD --> fumaric acid + FADH2 dehydrogenase

6) The formation of malic acid is the next step under the action of fumarate: smoke Fumaric acid + H2O -> malic acid The energy released in this reaction is small and therefore the reaction is irreversible.

7) The oxidation of malic acid to oxal-acetic acid is the last stage of the Krebs cycle under the action of malic-dehydrogenase. Through the Krebs cycle, complete oxidation of the acetyl radical to CO2 and H2O is achieved. malate Malic acid + NAD + -> oxal-acetic acid + NADH + H + ß --- dehydrogenase Δ Go = 7.1 kcal /mol.

The reaction is endogenous but the reaction is shifted to the right because both oxaloacetate and NADH2 are rapidly engaged in other processes. From a bioenergetic point of view, the whole process of aerobic degradation of glycolysis can be summarized as follows:

(Δ Go = - 57 kcal/mol)

The total energy balance of the Krebs cycle is 15 moles of ATP for each molecule of pyruvic acid. The Krebs cycle, beginning with the synthesis of citric acid, takes place in the inner compartment of the mitochondria, where the enzymes are located in the soluble matrix while others are bound to the inner mitochondrial membrane. A process of universality for all organisms is the oxidation of hydrogen contained in the organic molecules of the substrate by atmospheric oxygen with the formation of water and the release of energy. Substrate hydrogen is transferred to O2 via intermediate hydrogen and electron transporters, which are redox systems with increasing redox potential.

Each transported hydrogen atom releases 2e- from the components of the respiratory chain. Following the citrate cycle, 8 hydrogen atoms are transported through redox systems. When transferring 2e- on intermediate transports, the most common cause of biological oxidation reductions is an energy of 46.5 kcal/mol, at pH 7, which will be incorporated in 6 moles of ATP.

If the respiratory chain starts with NAD, there are three stages in which energy is released to form ATP; these steps are called phosphorylation steps. The ratio between the amount of bound phosphate in the form of ATP and the amount of O2 consumed during the development of the respiratory chain, respectively the P / O ratio is called "how much phosphorylation".

The global equation for the phosphorylation of a pyruvic acid molecule can be written as follows:

NADH + H + + 3ADP + 3Pi +1/2 O2 -> NAD + + 4H2O + 3ATP 2H + 1/2 O2 --> H2O

This is the equation of the formation of an H2O molecule to which that energy corresponds. The second equation is endergonic: 3ADP + 3Pi --> 3ATP + 3H2O Δ Go = 21 kcal / mol

From the energy of water formation, it is stored as biologically active energy, the energy corresponding to the formation of three molecules of ATP, so 3 x 7.8 kcal = 23.4 kcal. So, if 23.4 kcal were incorporated into ATP from 45 kcal, the process yield will be about 40.05%.

An increase in the concentration of ADP and phosphate leads to a strong intensification of oxidation processes (ex. muscle effort), while in the case of a very large increase in the concentration of ATP can even lead to a reversal of oxidative phosphorylation which means that respiratory control is installed through "energy hunger".

The fundamental process of energy conservation consists of a vector transport of H + from the matrix space of the mitochondria (M) through the mitochondrial membrane into the intermembrane space (C). This transport of protons creates an electrochemical gradient that stimulates ATP synthesis and oxidative phosphorylation, respectively.

Of the 8H transported along the respiratory chain, 6H is in the form of 3 NADH2 molecules with the formation of 9 molecules of ATP, and 2H is in the form of FADH2 which will give rise to another 2 molecules of ATP.

To this Krebs cycle, ATP balance has added the formation of an ATP molecule by phosphorylation of substances (conversion of succinyl CoA to succinate). Therefore, 12 molecules of ATP will be formed from the Krebs cycle to oxidize one molecule of pyruvic acid. By coupling the cycle with oxidative phosphorylation in the respiratory chain, 15 molecules of ATP will be formed.

Coupling the Krebs cycle with the respiratory chain in the mitochondria is the main source of biological energy for chemical-synthetic organisms. From a molecule of glucose, arising during its "aerobic degradation" two molecules of pyruvic acid means that 30 moles of ATP will form at the mitochondrial level. If we take into account the 8 molecules of cytoplasmic

ATP used during the glycolysis process, it means that by the complete degradation of one molecule of glucose, 38 molecules of ATP will be formed. The corresponding energy expressed in calories will be 299.06 kcal (38x7.8 k mol).

The energy-theoretical efficiency of the carbohydrate degradation process is approximately 43.5% because of the 686 kcal accumulated in the glucose molecule during the photosynthesis process, only 299.06 kcal are returned to the body by degrading carbohydrates. The exclusively aerobic energy yield of the mitochondria through the Krebs cycle for the glucose molecule will be around 41.05% because the 654.51 kcal that enters the aerobic cycle will result at the end of only 321.6 kcal of which 228 kcal represents only the energy of 4 molecules of water and 93.6 kcal of bioenergy stored in the 12 molecules of ATP (12x7.8 k mol).

CH3 - COOH + 2H2O + 2O2------> 2CO2 + 4H2O

The rest of the bioenergy is lost from reversible transfers. ATP phosphate couplings, therefore, serve to activate products by phosphorylation or as binding or recognition groups for substrate enzyme systems. Phosphorylation charges the reagent molecules negatively, which means blocking the free diffusion through the cell membranes of the reagents. Coupling enzymes with ATP and then with glucose for phosphorylation to initiate glycolysis requires the presence of Ca2 + and Mg2 + ions.

Animal tissue mitochondria can accumulate certain Ca2 + cations against the concentration gradient in an energetically coupled process with electron transport. Ca accumulation is accompanied by the consumption of equivalent amounts of phosphate. A pair of electrons moving through NADH2 to O2 accumulates an average of about six Ca2 + ions, two for each phosphorylation step. When Ca ions accumulate, oxidative phosphorylation no longer occurs, so the formation of ATP,

For every intramitochondrial transport Ca is an important factor in regulating the concentration of Ca2 + in the cytosol, on which many cellular activities depend. The cellular energy level is an important factor in the regulation of carbohydrate metabolic regulation processes. When the amount of intracellular ATP is low, the concentration of nitrate decreases, which causes the transient accumulation of acetyl-CoA which will stimulate pyruvate carboxylase. Oxaloacetate will focus on citrate formation because at low ATP concentrations citrate synthesis is very active.

When the ATP concentration is increased, gluconeogenesis conditions are created: citrate synthesis is inhibited and oxaloacetate does not bind to acetyl-CoA. Since acetyl-CoA cannot be directed to fatty acid synthesis (the reaction to form acetyl-CoA fatty acids requires citrate activation) it will activate pyruvate carboxylase, directing oxaloacetate to phosphoenolpyruvate synthesis and thus to glucose.

At very high concentrations of ATP, inhibition of phosphofructokinase, an aerobic glycolysis enzyme, which converts F-i-P to the reactive form F-6-P occurs. If we have a large amount of mitochondrial ATP in the cellular environment, the anaerobic glycolytic pathway is stopped, or inhibited, like long-molecule fatty acids or citrates. When in the environment we have high concentrations of ADP or AMP then phosphofructokinase is activated for the glycolytic pathway.

Also, the accumulation of ATP in the cell as a final product of the Krebs cycle and oxidative phosphorylation causes inhibition of the pyruvate dehydrogenase complex which converts pyruvic acid to acetyl CoA. The Pasteur effect is a mechanism for regulating energy consumption and occurs when energy consumption is low. Thus, the process of glycolysis that is not economically economical (produces only two moles of ATP / mol of glucose) is replaced by the process of respiration that has a higher energy efficiency (produces 38 moles of ATP / mol of glucose).

The Pasteur effect is not effective in lung tissue and tumor tissue where the presence of molecular O2 does not inhibit the glycolysis process. In the tumor tissue, the intensity of glycolysis in the presence of O2 is higher the more malignant the tumors. The growth of tumor cells could be explained by the change in the normal relationship between respiration and glycolysis.

In the metabolism of a healthy cell, in the presence of O2, the use of glycolysis is lower and the accumulation of lactic acid is more suppressed. The Pasteur effect, therefore, consists of an almost total inhibition of the lactic acid formation process and the orientation of the reactants towards the formation of CO2 and H2O, as final products, in the presence of O2.

Therefore, the glycolytic reaction is replaced by the oxidative degradation reaction, which is reduced to the inhibition of glycolysis by respiration. In the process of oxidative degradation, P and ADP, in the presence of O2, are removed from the glycolysis process, which they inhabit. At the same time, the inhibition of phosphofructokinase by citrate and the oxidation of SH

groups, essential for the-phosphate dehydrogenase, take place in the presence of O_2. The aerobic pathway can be inhibited by:

* stop the cellular respiration with specific toxins and carcinogens;
• inactivation of triose-phosphate dehydrogenases;
• decoupling of oxidative phosphorylation.

If glucose is added to normal or tum0r tissue, inhibition of O_2 consumption is observed, as inhibition of respiration by glycolysis or an inverted Pasteur effect (Crabtree effect). In this process, competition for inorganic phosphate predominates. The appearance of the Crabtree effect can be explained by a disorder in hexokinase, a phosphorylating enzyme for inorganic phosphate. Hexokinase is physiologically activated by normal insulin. Insulin also inhibits glucose-6-phosphatase, an enzyme that converts glucose-6-P m to free glucose. Due to the accumulation of ATP at the mitochondrial level, hexokinase located in the cytoplasm cannot exert its catabolic activity due to lack of ATP, and phosphorylation of glucose will be slow in anaerobiosis. The coupling of the catabolic processes with the anabolic ones is frequently achieved through ATP, the reservoir for the energy released during the catabolism and at the same time the supplier of the energy needed in the biosynthesis processes.

Glucose biosynthesis, in particular glucose-6-phosphate, can occur from carbohydrate or non-carbohydrate compounds. Glucose-6-phosphate can be formed in multiple ways:

a). by photosynthesis in green plants, then absorbed in the intestine;

b). by converting lactic acid to pyruvic acid into glucose;

c). by glycogenesis in the Krebs cycle intermediates;

d). by amino acid glycogenesis; e). by the conversion of other hexoses into glucose-6-phosphorus.

The process of glucose synthesis in green plants was described in the chapter "ATP - the universal energy reservoir". The conversion of pyruvic acid to glucose can be done in several stages: a) formation of phosphoenolpyruvate from pyruvic acid: b) Pyruvic acid + ATP -> phospho-enol-pyruvic acid ß, ($\Delta Go = 0.2$ kcal/mol). The above overall reaction indicates a small variation in free energy as two reactions are assumed to exist: The endergonic reaction is Pyruvic acid + GTP --> pyruvic acid phospho-enol ($\Delta Go = 1.7$ kcal/mol).

The exogenous reaction is:

ATP + H2O -> ADP + P2 (Δ Go = -7.3 kcal / mol)

The phosphorylation of pyruvate to phosphoenolpyruvate required energy from one molecule of ATP and one molecule of GTP. The resulting phosphoenolpyruvate is further converted to fructose-1-bisphosphate. Fructose-1-6, bisphosphate is formed under the action of phospho-fructo-kinase based on the reaction:

F-6-P + ATP -> F1,6-P + ADP
F1.6P + H2O -> F-6-P + P2 (Δ Go = 4.04 kcal / mol) ADP + Pi ->ATP ß -F-6-P --> G-6-P ß, reversible reaction

During glycolysis, G-6-P is formed by direct phosphorylation of glucose by ATP and in the presence of hexokinase. In anabolic reactions, the formation of free glucose takes place by the hydrolysis of G-6-P under the action of the enzyme G-6-phosphatase. G-6-P + H2O ---> G + P2 (ΔGo = -3.3 kcal/mol) This enzyme is selectively distributed in the endoplasmic reticulum of the liver and kidneys. G-6-phosphatase is not found in muscles and the brain, organs that cannot form free glucose. Glucose can also be formed by the Krebs cycle from amino acids: glycine, arginine, histidine, proline, hydroxyproline, cistern, tryptophan, etc. The main hexoses: glucose, fructose, galactose, and mannose, can be transformed into each other, depending on the need of the body at a given time:

Hexokinase Fructose + ATP --> F-6-P + ADP or fructokinase Fructose + ATP ---> F-l-P + ADP

The metabolic background of glucose required for active organs is achieved by the synthesis of glycogen in the case of excess free glucose and by the degradation of glycogen in the case of glucose deficiencies. The synthesis and degradation of glycogen concerning the needs of the body are regulated by various mechanisms based on the enzyme glycogen synthetase which ensures the synthesis of glycogen, as well as the enzyme phosphorylase which ensures its degradation.

These transformations take place with the participation of ATP and under the action of an activated cyclic AMP kinase. Thus, phosphorylase "b" (dimer) under the action of active phosphorylase-b-kinase with the participation of 4 molecules of ATP, passes into active phosphorylase "a" (tetramer) and catalyzes the degradation of glycogen. Conversely, inactive

glycogen synthesis undergoes dephosphorylation into active glycogen synthetase. The reaction is catalyzed by a specific kinase.

The two opposite processes are under hormonal and nervous control exerted by complex mechanisms involving cAMP. Carbohydrate energy has the advantage of being accessible, variable energy, and able to provide immediate but short-term energy needs during periods of high demand. Thus, glucose can be considered an immediate source of energy in the body as opposed to lipids which are a form of energy storage in the body. In mammals, it has been estimated that glucose is degraded 90% glycolytically.

The EMP pathway predominates massively, especially in muscles and the brain. In the muscles, carbohydrate degradation is the initial product of glycogen, as muscle fibre does not contain appreciable amounts of free glucose. At a moderate muscular effort, the degradation of glucose is done by the oxidation of pyruvic acid resulting from glycolysis using tricarboxylic acids. In an intense muscular effort, the degradation of glucose becomes anaerobic with the reduction of pyruvic acid to lactic acid and the accumulation of lactic acid proportional to the degree and duration of the effort.

At rest, when the O3 reserves are renewed, the lactic acid is re-oxidized under the action of the enzyme Lacto-dehydrogenase to pyruvic acid which, after its oxidative decarboxylation, enters the cycle of tricarboxylic acids. The ratio of glucose to respiration in facultative cells capable of degrading glucose in both ways is determined by the amount of O2 in the cell.

If oxidative decoupling by carcinogens occurs over time, their long-term action will result in increased glycolysis, the establishment of anaerobic metabolism, and the evolution of the cell along the path of cancer. The pathway of glucose degradation pentose-phosphates is uncommon. ATP is not formed in this way but, on the contrary, is consumed by the phosphorylation reactions of glucose.

The pentose-phosphate pathway is usually expressed more intensely in the metabolism of embryonic and neoplastic tissues or organs with an important role in the biosynthesis of nucleic acids, creating material for protein structural components or in the biosynthesis of fatty acids and sterol compounds. These include the liver, mammary gland, red blood cells (80% of glucose degradation is done in this way although they carry O2 embedded in hemoglobin), pancreas, thyroid, adrenal glands, kidneys, and leukocytes. In the following chapters, we will seek to deepen the mechanisms of cellular

bioenergetic potential that ensure the functionality of normal or malignant cells.

3. The role of the ATP complex in lipid metabolism

Lipids are a major source of energy for the body. To store 100 Kal you need 100 gr. of tissue in time for the same quantity of calories stored in the form of glycogen is needed 130 gr. of tissue. The catabolism of fatty acids is achieved through an oxidation process. Fatty acids are chemically inert, and activation is required to take part in the chain of oxidative degradation reactions.

This activation is performed in an initial step by coupling the fatty acids with HS CoA, through a thioester bond. In this coupling reaction, acyl CoA is formed which represents the activated substrate. The acyl-CoA formation reaction takes place in the presence of fatty acid and ATP. The high energy thioester bond of CoA arises from the conversion of ATP to AMP with the release of a pyrophosphoric acid molecule:

acyl CoA HS ~ CoA + ATP + R --> (CH2) n ------> COOH --> R- (CH2) n - synthetase -S + CoA + AMP + 2Pi (acyl CoA)

In this activated form of acyl-CoA, the fatty acid enters the chain of oxidative degradation reactions until the whole fatty acid molecule is transformed into acyl-CoA. For example, the degradation of a fatty acid with 16 C atoms (palmitic acid) will result in 8 molecules of acyl-CoA along with $FADH_2$ and $NADH_2$ with a gain of 360 moles of ATP per molecule of fatty acid. Degradation of each acetyl-CoA unit via the Krebs cycle releases 12 moles of ATP, so 96 moles of ATP will be released for the 8 molecules of acyl-CoA. Energy is released in a spiral in steps catalyzed by redox enzymes.

Going through a spiral releases 5 moles of ATP. The spiral is repeated by (n / 2 -1), where "n" is the number of C atoms in the acid molecule so that in the case of fatty acid with 16 C atoms the number of moles of ATP released by beta-oxidation will be equal with (16/2 -1) x 5 = 35 moles of ATP; 96 moles of ATP + 35 moles of ATP = 131 moles of ATP As only 1 mole of ATP is consumed in the degradation reaction, the net gain per molecule of fatty acid (palmitic) is therefore 130 moles of ATP.

Hence the energy importance of lipids for the body. The acyl-CoA formed cannot follow the path of ketone body formation in depletion quantities. Its

admission to the Krebs cycle is not possible due to the small amount of oxalate present as a result of the Krebs cycle at a very low rate, and the formation of fatty acids and steroid hormones from acetyl CoA requires NADPH resulting in the direct oxidation of ozone, disrupted and he in these conditions.

The prevention of ketosis is achieved by the so-called catalytic substances, represented by the Krebs acid substrate, by the fatty acid gluco-forming amino acids with an odd number of C atoms which by degradation give propionyl CoA convertible to succinyl CoA. ATP also initiates "de novo" fatty acid biosynthesis through a two-stage reaction: Stimulation of fatty acid biosynthesis by SH-substances and inhibition by SH-blocking factors show the role of these groups in fatty acid synthesis reactions. Neutral fats consist of glycerol and fatty acids and their catabolism includes degradation processes of each component.

Glycol catabolism is integrated into the carbohydrate degradation cycle with intermediate formation of glycerophosphate:

glycerol + ATP --> α glycerophosphate + ADP
glycerol-phosphokinase

This form of glycerol may be degraded by carbohydrate metabolism or may be incorporated into the body's synthesized fats. Choline and choline that participate in the synthesis of glycerol-phosphatides (lecithin and cephalins) take part in these reactions in their activated form. Their activation takes place in the presence of a specific cofactor: CTP, UTP and ATP. The intestinal mucosa ensures the resynthesis of triglycerides from two mono-acyls: glycerol and fatty acid. This process requires energy, namely: two molecules of ATP per mole of triacylglycerol.

The two molecules of ATP are used to activate fatty acids. Activation and penetration of fatty acids into the mitochondria takes place through a catalyzed reaction of ATP-dependent to-kinases. Fatty acids and glycerol, respectively, are important sources of energy in biological systems, due to their ability to oxidize completely to CO3 and H2O, thus releasing the entire amount of energy contained in their molecule. If the net amount of ATP that is formed by β - the oxidation of a fatty acid with 16 C atoms (palmitic) is 130 moles of ATP means that this amount is equivalent to 910 kcal incorporated.

The combustion heat of palmitic acid is 2340 kcal/mol, according to the equation:

CH3 - (CH2) 14 - COOH + 23 O2 --> 16 CO2 + 16 H2O

Therefore, of the 2340 kcal released after the complete oxidation of palmitic acid to CO2 and H2O, only 910 kcal are stored as ATP. The energy efficiency, in this case, is 38.8%. Thus, about 38% of the free oxidative energy of palmitic acid is recovered as energy in the macro-energic phosphate bonds in ATP. Extensive research by biochemists in recent times has shown that the "de novo" synthesis of fatty acids from precursors takes place in the soluble fraction of the cytoplasm and is catalyzed by a multienzyme system, consisting of a group of 7 enzymes.

This complex called acyl synthetase is stable and therefore difficult to dissociate in animal tissues. In the cytoplasm of animal cells, the biosynthesis of palmitic acid predominates, in this process, an acetyl CoA molecule serves as a "primer" or "starter", the subsequent fragments coming from the malonyl CoA molecule. The synthesis of palmitic acid can take place neither in the mitochondria nor in the endoplasmic reticulum, but in these cellular subfractions, the chain elongation of fatty acids that already contain 12-16 C atoms can take place.

The fundamental structural unit in fatty acid biosynthesis is ultimately intramitochondrial acetyl-CoA. In mitochondria, acetyl-CoA can result from two major processes: a) β - oxidation of fatty acids; b) decarboxylation of pyruvic acid. Because of this, acetyl-CoA first condenses into oxalyl-acetate to form citric acid, and citric acid passes easily from the mitochondria into the cytoplasm. In the cytoplasm, citric acid is further cleaved into acetyl-COA and oxalyl-acetate, the energy required for this process being provided by ATP.

Acetyl CoA carboxylation to malonyl CoA biotin takes place in the cytoplasm:

CH3-CO-SCOA + C02 + ATP -> HOOC-CH2 OSCOH + ADP + Pi Mn2

The malonyl CoA formation reaction is the soothing reaction of the whole sequence (pacemaker). Activation of acetyl CoA carboxylase is greatly enhanced by the presence of titrate and isocitrate which act as modulators of the carboxylation reaction. Glycerol-3-P can also be formed by the phosphorylation of free glycerol resulting from the hydrolysis of triacylglycerol:

Glycerol + ATP --> glycerol-3-P + ADP Glycerol-3-P is oxidized to hydroxy-acetone phosphate which enters the glycolytic pathway or the

synthesis of glycerol-phosphatides (phosphatidic acid). Another pathway of glycerol-phosphatide synthesis is based on the activation of nitrogen compounds by CTP, followed by the corresponding diacylglycerol reaction. Example:

Choline + ATP --> phosphocholine + ADP

The process of cholesterol biosynthesis takes place from simple molecules of active acetate or CH3-CO-SCOA, which through a series of intermediate steps form compounds with a higher number of C atoms. The sequence of reactions leading to cholesterol synthesis is as follows:

1) condensation of the acetyl molecule CoA;

2) reduction to mevalonic acid;

3) phosphorylation and decarboxylation of mevalonic acid in three successive phases: mevalonic acid --> phospho-mevalonic acid --> pyro-phospho-mevalonic acid --> unstable compound --> iso-pentyl-pyrophosphate --> squalene (cholesterol precursor);

4) squalene cyclization and transformation of lanosterol into cholesterol. All these steps require ATP which will be transformed into ADP, with the release of energy required for each step. The level of cholesterol synthesis is generally influenced by the presence of important factors that participate in the mentioned stages: CoA, NADH, NADPH, and ATP.

Some of these compounds are formed in carbohydrate metabolism (NADH, NADPH, ATP). Thus, disorders of this metabolism also influence the process of cholesterol biosynthesis. The transformation of cholesterol into bile acids is the major route of cholesterol catabolism in mammals and occurs mainly in the liver.

Cholesterol, by oxidation and hydroxylation, is converted to cholic acid. Cholic acid in the presence of ATP and CoA changes to colyl-CoA which can be conjugated to glycine or taurine to form glyco-cholic or taurocholic acid. In the intestine, bile salts play an important role in the process of digestion and absorption. The metabolism of various categories of lipids has Ioc in most organs and tissues and is conditioned by numerous neuroendocrine factors.

The pathological changes of lipid metabolism are correlated with those of carbohydrate metabolism depending on the functional state of the main

organs involved in the metabolism of these compounds. Thus, diabetes significantly alters not only carbohydrate and lipid metabolism. Atherosclerosis involves profound changes in all categories of lipids. Acute and chronic hepatitis, pancreatitis of various types, nephrotic syndrome, pituitary dysfunction, and obesity cause strong changes in the metabolism of the main categories of tissue lipids: triglycerides, fatty acids (ag), cholesterol, etc. It has been found that overweight people have a higher proportion of cancer deaths than weak people (in 68% of cases):

Citrate + ATP + HS - CoA ------> acetyl CoA + ADP + Pi + oxal-lactate

Under experimental conditions, decreasing the intake of hydrocarbons (carbohydrates) in the diet, it was observed the delay in inducing tumors in guinea pigs. A vitamin-deficient diet reduces the activity of metabolic enzymes. In conclusion, I emphasize that the rational regime of life can oppose the establishment of malignant tum0ur metabolism in the apparatus and systems of the human body.

The overall picture of urea biosynthesis is as follows: In the muscular system, creatine reacts with ATP formed during glucose metabolism, which forms phosphocreatine, a macro-ergic compound: creatine + ATP -- phosphocreatine + ADP In muscle, phosphocreatine acts as a macro-organic phosphate reservoir. During muscle contraction, there is a significant consumption of ATP which is the direct source of energy of muscle contraction. ATP regenerates rapidly due to phosphocreatine as follows: PC + ADP -> creatine + ATP Therefore, phosphocreatine in muscle is an indirect source of energy consumed in muscle contraction. In muscle tissue, there is a balance between the processes that generate ATP molecules and the processes that consume ATP. Excess ATP results in a regeneration of phosphocreatine and increased ATP intake is affected by ATP-synthesizing systems.

In this way, a reserve of connections with high energy potential is maintained. Glycogen is the primary energy source of muscle tissue, and ATP - is the immediate and directly accessible energy source. Phosphocreatine, (FC), is an energy reservoir accessible only by ATP - the specific acceptor for the phosphate group - with ADP being dissolved.

FC + ADP -> creatine + ATP ß, (reversible reaction)
2ADP --> ATP + AMP
AMP ---> IMP --> deamination.

The state of relaxation of a muscle is determined by a high ATP content associated with poor ATPase enzyme activity. ATP hydrolyzed under the action of shrinkage actomyosin justifies discontinuation of contraction as a result of a competitive process between the relaxing and the shrinking effect. The grouping of SH in myosin by its blocking action prevents the binding and cleavage of ATP molecules. In the ossification process, ATP releases pyrophosphoric acid which combines with the bone matrix and remains bound to the collagen of the matrix by polar groups.

At the renal level, in the process of tubular resorption, the substances with high active threshold resorbed and saved by the body: glucose, amino acids, vitamin C, uric acid, Na, Ca, Mg, P and S is made by an active process against the gradient of concentration due to the energy intake of ATP and specific enzymatic mechanisms. Glutathione is synthesized in the body through a process that takes place in two stages and in which glycocol also participates. A glutamine-cysteine dipeptide is formed from glutamic acid and cysteine. Glutamine-cysteine is synthesized with glycochol to give rise to a tripeptide called glutathione. Both reactions require the presence of ATP and Mg in the second stage.

Condensation of glycol with benzoic acid, which is toxic to the body, forms hippuric acid, a non-toxic substance: Threonine is a gluco-forming amino acid that starts its biosynthesis from aspartic acid with the consumption of 2ATP and the participation of NADP. In the carboxylation stage of leucine, hydroxymethyl-glutamine CoA is formed, an important compound in protein metabolism. The activation reaction is a complex endergonic process that requires the presence of activated CO2 and is performed in the presence of a biotin enzyme and ATP as an energy donor. In transmethylation processes, methionine activation is an enzymatic process that requires the presence of Mg and reduced glutathione. The reaction takes place in the presence of ATP which, by dissolving three molecules of phosphoric acid, releases the adenosyl radical which binds to the sulfur atom in the methionine molecule:

methionine + ATP ------> CH3 - S - adenosylmethionine + H3PO4

The energy of the macro-ergic phosphate bonds in ATP is transferred to the methyl bile group. Upon activation, methionine in the form of adenosine

methionine participates in a series of transmethylation reactions on specific acceptors (norepinephrine --> adrenaline). The biosynthesis of coenzymes with nucleotide structure, in which the participation of nucleotides is necessary, is done with the help of nucleotide triphosphates, especially with the participation of ATP.

A category of coenzymes comes from vitamins, especially from the B group of vitamins. Thus, riboflavin (vitamin B2) can be phosphorylated to form flavin-nucleotide (FMN) or riboflavin monophosphate.

Riboflavin -- ATP --> FMN + ADP

FMN can react with another molecule of ATP to form FAD, (flavin-adenine-nucleotide): FMN + ATP ------> FAD + PP2. The structure of NAD and NADP is also a nucleotide structure. Coenzyme A also has a partial nucleotide structure and its biosynthesis requires the participation of ATP. The structure of vitamin B12 also recognizes a fragment with a nucleotide structure consisting of dimethyl-benzidine-imidazole, pentose, and phosphoric acid. ATP is also involved in activating other vitamins to convert them to coenzymes or enzymes. This is the case with thiamine, pyridoxal, biotin, and lipoic acid. The reactions are as follows:

Thiamine + ATP -> Thiamine-PPi, (Pyridoxal), + AMP

Pyridoxal + ATP --> Pyridoxal-P +

Biotin + ATP --> Biotin-adenine + PPi

Biotin-adenine + enzyme --> Biotin-enzyme + AMP

Lipoate + ATP - -> Lipoate-adenylate + PPi

It has been found that enzymes called DNA polymerases (I, II, III) and ligases are involved in DNA biosynthesis. DNA polymerase is mainly involved in the repair of modified DNA under the influence of various factors. The main features of the process are:

a). the corresponding nucleoside triphosphates, mono and inactive diphosphates are involved in the reactions, which means that high energy is required to carry out this process;

b). for the reaction to take place, the presence of all four nucleotide triphosphates (ATP, GTP, CTP, TTP) is required; the absence of one of them implies polycondensation

c). the reaction depends on the presence of Mg + ions;

d). a preformed DNA is required to carry out the reaction;

e). The DNA-RNA system reaction also has a nucleophilic mechanism by which the nucleophilic 3-OH group binds to the phosphoryl group in the nucleotide triphosphate releasing pyrophosphate. DNA ligases complement the action of polymerases allowing the creation of 3'-5 'diester bonds on which the formation of a circular molecular bond is initiated.

The action of DNA ligases requires the participation of ATP as well as other factors: - in tumor cells the transcription has from RNA-DNA-RNA under the action of reverse polymerase DNA polymerase-transcriptase;

- DNA biosynthesis could be determined by highlighting 9x104 intra-nucleotide bonds per minute. Frequently the cell can "repair" the altered nucleic acid under the action of endonucleases. Through these enzymes, the modified fragment is removed from the nucleic acid molecule, and under the action of DNA polymerases a direct nucleotide fragment is introduced, the process being controlled by the pre-existing matrix DNA in the cell.

Changes in the structure of DNA, the carrier of genetic information, can occur in larger portions, leading to changes in the structure of the reproductive process. At the same time, ATP is an activator of allosteric enzymes. In some enzymes, enzymatic phosphorylation results in their activation or inactivation. Glutamine synthetase consists of 12 units that modify their activity by introducing a residue of AMP from ATP into each of the 12 subunits and thus inactivates. In the case of glutamine synthetase, the activation of the enzyme takes place through a process of phosphorylase.

Transferases are a class of enzymes that catalyze a reaction such as R - A + R '- B ----------> R - B' + R '- A wherein part of the molecule of a substrate called a donor is transferred to another layer called an acceptor:

a). Trans-methylases are a class of enzymes that transfer the methyl group from the donor to the acceptor according to the reaction: R - CH3 + R '- H ---> R - H + R' - CH3 ß.

The transformation of the apparent donor substrate into the actual donor substrate is done by oxidation reaction or by charging with the energy released by ATP. Example: ATP + methionine ---> S - adenosylmethionine ß -+ H3PO4

b). trans-acetylase transfers acyl groups (acyl residues) from donors to receptors. Activation of organic acids by their transformation into acyl-CoA derivatives is done by providing ATP. The overall acetic acid activation reaction can be formulated as follows:

CH3 - COOH + CoA: SH + ATP ----> CH3 - CO ~ S - CoA + AMP + PPi Acetic acid ß ---- CoA acid.

The reactions are catalyzed by specific enzymes in the liver and other tissues. Nucleotide phosphorylases catalyze the transfer reaction of the residue of ribose 1-phosphate from ribose 1,5-bisphosphate to adenine, with nucleotide formation: **ribose - 1.5 diphosphate + adenine -------> AMP + H3PO4 ß**

Phosphokinases catalyze the general reaction: ATP + X ------> ADP + X-P

These enzymes play an important role in biosynthetic processes because they allow the release of energy accumulated in the macro-energetic phosphate bonds in the ATP molecule. Among the most important phosphokinases are:

a) hexokinase b) phosphokinases;

c) tri-phospho-glycerol-kinases; d) pyruvate kinase; e) myokinase; f) creatine kinase; g) nucleotide diphospho-kinases. Nucleotide di-phosphokinase catalyzes the transfer of phosphate from ATP to UDP (uridine-phosphate) or IDP (inosine in-phosphate) after reactions:

UDP + ATP --> UTP + ADP IDP + ATP -> ITP + ADP

Biotin plays an important role in carboxylation-decarboxylation reactions. Decarboxylation enzymes require the presence of ATP for their activity: ATP + biotin enzyme --> ADP biotin enzyme + H3PO4 This complex reacts with CO2 which, by substituting ADP, forms a new CO2 complex - the biotin enzyme.

This pasture elates the macro-energic bond and represents an activated CO2 capable of participating in carboxylation reactions: ADP - biotin enzyme + CO2 -> CO2 – biotin-enzyme + ADP Ligases, known as synthetases, catalyze the formation of a bond between two molecules in the presence of ATP as an energy donor.

X + Y + ATP --> X - Y + ATP + PPi ß, (reversible reaction)

Among the most important ligases are carboxylases that act on the type of reaction:

R - H + CO2 + H2O + ATP --> R - COOH + ADP + Pi ß.

DNA topoisomerase, recently discovered as a malignancy factor, is 20 times higher in cancer cells than in normal cells. This enzyme helps in the transcription of malignant DNA in very large quantities. Research continues. Biotin is a B-complex vitamin and acts as a coenzyme, a carrier of CO2 during the carboxylation process that can be released in biosynthesis processes on acceptor pyruvate:

Acetic acid + CO2 + ATP + H2O --> oxalyl-acetic acid carboxylase

The energy resulting from the degradation of large biomolecules to small molecules can be used at least partially in biosynthetic processes after its prior storage in compounds containing macro-ergic bonds.

Through their hydrolysis, the biochemical energy necessary for the biosynthesis of various natural organic compounds is formed, as they are consumed, formed and then regenerated during metabolic processes, thus fulfilling the role of coenzymes in addition to enzymes called kinases. Coenzyme A consists of a phosphorylated ATP residue, a pantothenic acid residue and a cysteine residue.

Its function is based on the ability of the SH group of cysteamine to bind through macro-energic thioester bonds, acyl radicals in general, and especially acetyl radicals, which can be transferred during metabolism to appropriate receptors. Thiamine pyrophosphate is derived from the phosphorylation of thiamine with ATP and is the coenzyme of the processes of decarboxylation of aceto-acids, trans-acetylation, and phospho-acetylation. pyruvate decarboxylase Pyruvic acid --> acetic aldehyde then PP From the above we can conclude that ATP performs a transfer of functional groups. It contains two macro-energic bonds, the hydrolysis of which results in the energy required for endergonic biosynthetic processes.

Phosphate groups in the ATP molecule can be cleaved gradually or completely, by hydrolysis of ATP to result in ADP, AMP, adenosine and phosphate (Pi) or pyrophosphate (PPi) ions. ATP resynthesis takes place due to the energy resulting from tissue respiration, aerobic degradation of glucose, oxidation of fatty acids, etc. The cleavage of ATP into ADP + Pi is done by ATPase, and the released energy is usually used to activate a substrate to be activated. Following the interaction of ATP with GDP, GTP

and ADP will form, and under the action of a guanylate-cyclase from GTP, cGMP can form, which, like cAMP, acts as a mediator of the action of certain categories of hormones. The set of ATP converted to cAMP by an adenyl cyclase with cGMP will give rise to a permanent cellular bioenergetic reflux that underlies cell life.

The major energy source of the cell is the oxidation of the substrates of food principles in O2 from the air, transported by the blood to the tissues. The living cell obtains its energy by oxidizing the hydrogen released from the organic substrate processed by the body, the formation of CO2 appears as a secondary phenomenon, often dependent only indirectly on oxidation reactions, which ultimately lead to decarboxylation. Numerous unknowns and many uncertainties over the years of medical research have made it almost impossible to delineate the preclinical phase of chronic disease from the initial state of health. The detection of biochemical changes in the body's apparatus and systems before their clinical expression has been quite uncertain through investigations conducted with the usual paraclinical means, [3].

When the ATP concentration is increased, gluconeogenesis conditions are created: citrate-synthesis is inhibited and oxaloacetate does not bind to acetyl-CoA. Since acetyl-CoA cannot be directed to fatty acid synthesis (the reaction to form acetyl-CoA fatty acids requires citrate activation) it will activate pyruvate carboxylase, directing oxaloacetate to phosphoenolpyruvate synthesis and thus to glucose.

At very high concentrations of ATP, inhibition of phosphofructokinase, an aerobic glycolysis enzyme, which converts F-i-P to the reactive form F-6-P occurs. If we have a large amount of mitochondrial ATP in the cellular environment, the anaerobic glycolytic pathway is stopped, inhibited, like long-molecule fatty acids or citrates. When in the environment we have high concentrations of ADP or AMP then phosphofructokinase is activated for the glycolytic pathway.

Also, the accumulation of ATP in the cell as a final product of the Krebs cycle and oxidative phosphorylation causes inhibition of the pyruvate dehydrogenase complex which converts pyruvic acid to acetyl CoA. The Pasteur effect is a mechanism for regulating energy consumption and occurs when energy consumption is low. Thus, the process of glycolysis that is not economically economical (produces only two moles of ATP / mol of glucose) is replaced by the process of respiration that has a higher energy efficiency (produces 38 moles of ATP / mol of glucose).

The Pasteur effect is not effective in lung tissue and tumor tissue where the presence of molecular O_2 does not inhibit the glycolysis process. In the tumor tissue, the intensity of glycolysis in the presence of O_2 is higher the more malignant the tumors. The growth of tumor cells could be explained by the change in the normal relationship between respiration and glycolysis.

In the metabolism of a healthy cell, in the presence of O_2, the use of glycolysis is lower and the accumulation of lactic acid is more suppressed. The Pasteur effect therefore consists of an almost total inhibition of the lactic acid formation process and the orientation of the reactants towards the formation of CO_2 and H_2O, as final products, in the presence of O_2.

Therefore, glycolytic reaction is replaced by the oxidative degradation reaction, which is reduced to an inhibition of glycolysis by respiration. In the process of oxidative degradation, P and ADP, in the presence of O_2, are removed from the glycolysis process, which they inhibit. At the same time, the inhibition of phosphofructokinase by citrate and the oxidation of SH groups, essential for thri-phosphate dehydrogenase, take place in the presence of O_2. The aerobic pathway can be inhibited by:

* stopping the cellular respiration with specific toxins, carcinogens;
• inactivation of triose-phosphate dehydrogenases;
• decoupling of oxidative phosphorylation.

If glucose is added to normal or tumor tissue, an inhibition of O_2 consumption is observed, an inhibition of respiration by glycolysis or an inverted Pasteur effect (Crabtre effect). In this process, competition for inorganic phosphate predominates. The appearance of the Crabtree effect can be explained by a disorder in hexokinase, a phosphorylating enzyme for inorganic phosphate. Hexokinase is physiologically activated by normal insulin. Insulin also inhibits glucose-6-phosphatase, an enzyme that converts glucose-6-P m to free glucose. Due to the accumulation of ATP at the mitochondrial level, hexokinase located in the cytoplasm cannot exert its catabolic activity due to lack of ATP, and phosphorylation of glucose will be slow in anaerobiosis. The coupling of the catabolic processes with the anabolic ones is frequently achieved through ATP, the reservoir for the energy released during the catabolism and at the same time the supplier of the energy needed in the biosynthesis processes.

Glucose biosynthesis, in particular glucose-6-phosphate, can occur from carbohydrate or non-carbohydrate compounds. Glucose-6-phosphate can be formed in multiple ways:

a). by photosynthesis in green plants, then absorbed in the intestine;

b). by converting lactic acid to pyruvic acid into glucose;

c). by glycogenesis in the Krebs cycle intermediates;

d). by amino acid glycogenesis; e). by the conversion of other hexoses into glucose-6-phosphorus.

The process of glucose synthesis in green plants was described in the chapter "ATP - the universal energy reservoir". The conversion of pyruvic acid to glucose can be done in several stages: a) formation of phosphoenolpyruvate from pyruvic acid: b) Pyruvic acid + ATP -> phospho-enol-pyruvic acid ⇓, (Δ Go = 0.2 kcal / mol). The above overall reaction indicates a small variation in free energy as two reactions are assumed to exist: The endergonic reaction is: Pyruvic acid + GTP --> pyruvic acid phospho-enol (Δ Go = 1.7 kcal / mol).

The exogenous reaction is:

ATP + H2O -> ADP + P2 (ΔGo = -7.3 kcal / mol)

The phosphorylation of pyruvate to phosphoenolpyruvate required energy from one molecule of ATP and one molecule of GTP. The resulting phosphoenolpyruvate is further converted to fructose-1-bisphosphate. Fructose-1-6, bisphosphate is formed under the action of phospho-fructo-kinase based on the reaction:

F-6-P + ATP -> F1,6-P + ADP
F1.6P + H2O -> F-6-P + P2 (Δ Go = 4.04 kcal / mol) ADP + Pi ->ATP ⇓
-F-6-P --> G-6-P ⇓, reversible reaction

During glycolysis, G-6-P is formed by direct phosphorylation of glucose by ATP and in the presence of hexokinase. In anabolic reactions, the formation of free glucose takes place by the hydrolysis of G-6-P under the action of the enzyme G-6-phosphotase. G-6-P + H2O ---> G + P2 (ΔGo = -3.3 kcal / mol) This enzyme is selectively distributed in the endoplasmic reticulum of the liver and kidneys. G-6-phosphatase is not found in muscles and the brain, organs that do not have the ability to form free glucose. Glucose can also be formed by the Krebs cycle from amino acids: glycine, arginine, histidine, proline, hydroxyproline, cistern, tryptophan, etc. The main hexoses - glucose, fructose, galactose, and mannose - can be transformed into each other, depending on the need of the body at a given time:

Hexokinase Fructose + **ATP --> F-6-P + ADP or fructokinase Fructose + ATP ---> F-l-P + ADP**

The metabolic background of glucose required for active organs is achieved by the synthesis of glycogen in the case of excess free glucose and by the degradation of glycogen in the case of glucose deficiencies. The synthesis and degradation of glycogen in relation to the needs of the body are regulated by various mechanisms based on the enzyme glycogen synthetase which ensures the synthesis of glycogen, as well as the enzyme phosphorylase which ensures its degradation.

These transformations take place with the participation of ATP and under the action of an activated cyclic AMP kinase. Thus, phosphorylase "b" (dimer) under the action of active phosphorylase-b-kinase with the participation of 4 molecules of ATP, passes into active phosphorylase "a" (tetramer) and catalyzes the degradation of glycogen. Conversely, inactive glycogen synthesis undergoes dephosphorylation into active glycogen synthetase. The reaction is catalyzed by a specific kinase.

The two opposite processes are under hormonal and nervous control exerted by complex mechanisms involving cAMP. Carbohydrate energy has the advantage of being accessible, variable energy, able to provide immediate but short-term energy needs during periods of high demand. Thus, glucose can be considered an immediate source of energy in the body as opposed to lipids which are a form of energy storage of the body. In mammals, it has been estimated that glucose is degraded 90% glycolytically.

The EMP pathway predominates massively especially in muscles and brain. In the muscles, carbohydrate degradation is the initial product of glycogen, as muscle fiber does not contain appreciable amounts of free glucose. At a moderate muscular effort, the degradation of glucose is done by the oxidation of pyruvic acid resulting from glycolysis by means of tricarboxylic acids. In an intense muscular effort, the degradation of glucose becomes anaerobic with the reduction of pyruvic acid to lactic acid and the accumulation of lactic acid proportional to the degree and duration of the effort.

At rest, when the $O3$ reserves are renewed, the lactic acid is re-oxidized under the action of the enzyme lacto-dehydrogenase to pyruvic acid which, after its oxidative decarboxylation, enters the cycle of tricarboxylic acids. The ratio of glucose to respiration in facultative cells capable of degrading glucose in both ways is determined by the amount of O_2 in the cell.

If oxidative decoupling by carcinogens occurs over time, their long-term action will result in increased glycolysis, the establishment of anaerobic metabolism, and the evolution of the cell along the path of cancer. The pathway of glucose degradation pentose-phosphates is uncommon. ATP is not formed in this way but, on the contrary, is consumed by the phosphorylation reactions of glucose.

The pentose-phosphate pathway is usually expressed more intensely in the metabolism of embryonic and neoplastic tissues or in organs with an important role in the biosynthesis of nucleic acids, creating material for protein structural components or in the biosynthesis of fatty acids and sterol compounds. These include: liver, mammary gland, red blood cells (80% of glucose degradation is done in this way although they carry $O2$ embedded in hemoglobin), pancreas, thyroid, adrenal glands, kidneys, leukocytes. In the following chapters we will seek to deepen the mechanisms of cellular bioenergetic potential that ensure the functionality of normal or malignant cells.

4. The role of the ATP complex in lipid metabolism

Lipids are a major source of energy for the body. To store 100 kal you need 100 gr. of tissue in time for the same quantity of calories stored in the form of glycogen is needed 130 gr. of tissue. The catabolism of fatty acids is achieved through an oxidation process. Fatty acids have been shown to be chemically inert, and activation is required to take part in the chain of oxidative degradation reactions.

This activation is performed in an initial step by coupling the fatty acids with HS CoA, through a thioester bond. In this coupling reaction acyl CoA is formed which represents the activated substrate. The acyl-CoA formation reaction takes place in the presence of fatty acid and ATP. The high energy thioester bond of CoA arises from the conversion of ATP to AMP with the release of a pyrophosphoric acid molecule:

acyl CoA HS ~ CoA + ATP + R --> (CH2) n ------> COOH --> R- (CH2) n - synthetase -S + CoA + AMP + 2Pi (acyl CoA)

In this activated form of acyl-CoA the fatty acid enters the chain of oxidative degradation reactions until the whole fatty acid molecule is transformed into acyl-CoA. For example, the degradation of a fatty acid with 16 C atoms (palmitic acid) will result in 8 molecules of acyl-CoA along with FADH2 and NADH2 with a gain of 360 moles of ATP per molecule of fatty acid.

Degradation of each acetyl-CoA unit via the Krebs cycle releases 12 moles of ATP, so 96 moles of ATP will be released for the 8 molecules of acyl-CoA. Energy is released in a spiral in steps catalyzed by redox enzymes.

Going through a spiral releases 5 moles of ATP. The spiral is repeated by (n / 2 -1), where "n" is the number of C atoms in the acid molecule so that in the case of fatty acid with 16 C atoms the number of moles of ATP released by beta-oxidation will be equal with (16/2 -1) x 5 = 35 moles of ATP; 96 moles of ATP + 35 moles of ATP = 131 moles of ATP As only 1 mole of ATP is consumed in the degradation reaction, the net gain per molecule of fatty acid (palmitic) is therefore 130 moles of ATP.

Hence the energy importance of lipids for the body. The acyl-CoA formed cannot follow the path of ketone body formation in depletion quantities. Its admission to the Krebs cycle is not possible due to the small amount of oxalate present as a result of the Krebs cycle at a very low rate, and the formation of fatty acids and steroid hormones from acetyl CoA requires NADPH resulting in direct oxidation of ozone, disrupted and he in these conditions.

The prevention of ketosis is achieved by the so-called catalytic substances, represented by the Krebs acid substrate, by the fatty acid gluco-forming amino acids with an odd number of C atoms which by degradation give propionyl CoA convertible to succinyl CoA. ATP also initiates "de novo" fatty acid biosynthesis through a two-stage reaction: Stimulation of fatty acid biosynthesis by SH-substances and inhibition by SH-blocking factors show the role of these groups in fatty acid synthesis reactions. Neutral fats consist of glycerol and fatty acids and their catabolism includes degradation processes of each component.

Glycol catabolism is integrated into the carbohydrate degradation cycle with intermediate formation of glycerophosphate:

glycerol + ATP --> α glycerophosphate + ADP
glycerol-phosphokinase

This form of glycerol may be degraded by carbohydrate metabolism or may be incorporated into the body's synthesized fats. Choline and cholamine that participate in the synthesis of glycero-phosphatides (lecithin and cephalins) take part in these reactions in their activated form. Their activation takes place in the presence of a specific cofactor: CTP, UTP and ATP. The intestinal mucosa ensures the resynthesis of triglycerides from two mono-

acyls: glycerol and fatty acid. This process requires energy, namely: two molecules of ATP per mole of triacylglycerol.

The two molecules of ATP are used to activate fatty acids. Activation and penetration of fatty acids into the mitochondria takes place through a catalyzed reaction of ATP-dependent tio-kinases. Fatty acids and thri-glycerol, respectively, are important sources of energy in biological systems, due to their ability to oxidize completely to CO_3 and H_2O, thus releasing the entire amount of energy contained in their molecule. If the net amount of ATP that is formed by β - oxidation of a fatty acid with 16 C atoms (palmitic) is 130 moles of ATP means that this amount is equivalent to 910 kcal incorporated.

The combustion heat of palmitic acid is 2340 kcal / mol, according to the equation:

$$CH_3 - (CH_2)_{14} - COOH + 23\ O_2 \rightarrow 16\ CO_2 + 16\ H_2O$$

Therefore, of the 2340 kcal released after complete oxidation of palmitic acid to CO_2 and H_2O, only 910 kcal are stored as ATP. The energy efficiency in this case is 38.8%. Thus, about 38% of the free oxidative energy of palmitic acid is recovered as energy in the macro-energic phosphate bonds in ATP. Extensive research by biochemists in recent times has shown that the "de novo" synthesis of fatty acids from precursors takes place in the soluble fraction of the cytoplasm and is catalyzed by a multienzyme system, consisting of a group of 7 enzymes.

This complex called acyl synthetase is stable and therefore difficult to dissociate in animal tissues. In the cytoplasm of animal cells, the biosynthesis of palmitic acid predominates, in this process an acetyl CoA molecule serving as a "primer" or "starter", the subsequent fragments coming from the malonyl CoA molecule. The synthesis of palmitic acid can take place neither in the mitochondria nor in the endoplasmic reticulum, but in these cellular subfractions the chain elongation of fatty acids that already contain 12-16 C atoms can take place.

The fundamental structural unit in fatty acid biosynthesis is ultimately intramitochondrial acetyl-CoA. In mitochondria acetyl-CoA can result from two major processes: a) β - oxidation of fatty acids; b) decarboxylation of pyruvic acid. Because of this, acetyl-CoA first condenses into oxalyl-acetate to form citric acid, and citric acid passes easily from the mitochondria into the cytoplasm. In the cytoplasm, citric acid is further cleaved into acetyl-

COA and oxalyl-acetate, the energy required for this process being provided by ATP.

Acetyl CoA carboxylation to malonyl CoA biotin takes place in the cytoplasm:

CH3-CO-SCOA + C02 + ATP -> HOOC-CH2 OSCOH + ADP + Pi Mn2

The malonyl CoA formation reaction is in fact the soothing reaction of the whole sequence (pace-maker). Activation of acetyl CoA carboxylase is greatly enhanced by the presence of titrate and isocitrate which act as modulators of the carboxylation reaction. Glycerol-3-P can also be formed by phosphorylation of free glycerol resulting from the hydrolysis of triacylglycerol:

Glycerol + ATP --> glycerol-3-P + ADP Glycerol-3-P is oxidized to hydroxy-acetone phosphate which enters the glycolytic pathway or the synthesis of glycero-phosphatides (phosphatidic acid). Another pathway of glycero-phosphatide synthesis is based on the activation of nitrogen compounds by CTP, followed by the corresponding diacylglycerol reaction. Example:

Choline + ATP --> phosphocholine + ADP

The process of cholesterol biosynthesis takes place from simple molecules of active acetate or CH3-CO-SCOA, which through a series of intermediate steps form compounds with a higher number of C atoms. The sequence of reactions leading to cholesterol synthesis is as follows:

1) condensation of the acetyl molecule CoA;

2) reduction to mevalonic acid;

3) phosphorylation and decarboxylation of mevalonic acid in three successive phases: mevalonic acid --> phospho-mevalonic acid --> pyro-phospho-mevalonic acid --> unstable compound --> iso-pentyl-pyrophosphate --> squalene (cholesterol precursor);

4) squalene cyclization and transformation of lanosterol into cholesterol. All these steps require ATP which will be transformed into ADP, with the release of energy required for each step. The level of cholesterol synthesis is generally influenced by the presence of important factors that participate in the mentioned stages: CoA, NADH, NADPH, ATP.

Some of these compounds are formed in carbohydrate metabolism (NADH, NADPH, ATP). Thus, disorders of this metabolism also influence the process of cholesterol biosynthesis. The transformation of cholesterol into bile acids is the major route of cholesterol catabolism in mammals and occurs mainly in the liver.

Cholesterol, by oxidation and hydroxylation, is converted to cholic acid. Cholic acid in the presence of ATP and CoA changes to colyl-CoA which can be conjugated to glycine or taurine to form glyco-cholic or taurocholic acid. In the intestine, bile salts play an important role in the process of digestion and absorption. The metabolism of various categories of lipids has place in most organs and tissues and is conditioned by numerous neuroendocrine factors.

The pathological changes of lipid metabolism are correlated with those of carbohydrate metabolism depending on the functional state of the main organs involved in the metabolism of these compounds. Thus, diabetes significantly alters not only carbohydrate and lipid metabolism. Atherosclerosis involves profound changes in all categories of lipids. Acute and chronic hepatitis, pancreatitis of various types, nephrotic syndrome, pituitary dysfunction, obesity cause strong changes in the metabolism of the main categories of tissue lipids: triglycerides, fatty acids (ag), cholesterol, etc. It has been found that overweight people have a higher proportion of cancer deaths than weak people (in 68% of cases):

Citrate + ATP + HS - CoA ------> acetyl CoA + ADP + Pi + oxal-lactate

Under experimental conditions, by decreasing the intake of hydrocarbons (carbohydrates) in the diet, the delay in inducing tumors in guinea pigs was observed. A vitamin-deficient diet reduces the activity of metabolic enzymes. In conclusion, I emphasize that the rational regime of life can oppose the establishment of malignant tumor metabolism in the apparatus and systems of the human body.

The overall picture of urea biosynthesis is as follows: In the muscular system, creatine reacts with ATP formed during glucose metabolism, which forms phosphocreatine, a macro-ergic compound: creatine + ATP -- phosphocreatine + ADP In muscle, phosphocreatine acts as a macro-ergic phosphate reservoir. During muscle contraction there is a significant consumption of ATP which is the direct source of energy of muscle contraction. ATP regenerates rapidly due to phosphocreatine as follows: PC + ADP -> creatine + ATP Therefore, phosphocreatine in muscle is an

indirect source of energy consumed in muscle contraction. In muscle tissue there is a balance between the processes that generate ATP molecules and the processes that consume ATP. Excess ATP results in a regeneration of phosphocreatine and increased ATP intake is affected by ATP-synthesizing systems.

In this way, a reserve of connections with high energy potential is maintained. Glycogen is the primary energy source of muscle tissue, and ATP - the immediate and directly accessible energy source. Phosphocreatine, (FC), is an energy reservoir accessible only by ATP - the specific acceptor for the phosphate group - dissolved being ADP.

FC + ADP -> creatine + ATP ⇓, (reversible reaction)
2ADP --> ATP + AMP
AMP ---> IMP --> deamination.

The state of relaxation of a muscle is determined by a high ATP content associated with poor ATP-ase enzyme activity. ATP hydrolyzed under the action of shrinkage actomyosin justifies discontinuation of contraction as a result of a competitive process between the relaxing and the shrinking effect. The grouping of SH in myosin by its blocking action prevents the binding and cleavage of ATP molecules. In the ossification process, ATP releases pyrophosphoric acid which combines with the bone matrix and remains bound to the collagen of the matrix by polar groups.

At the renal level, in the process of tubular resorption, the substances with high active threshold resorbed and saved by the body: glucose, amino acids, vitamin C, uric acid, Na, Ca, Mg, P and S is made by an active process against the gradient of concentration due to the energy intake of ATP and specific enzymatic mechanisms. Glutathione is synthesized in the body through a process that takes place in two stages and in which glycocol also participates. Glutamine-cysteine dipeptide is formed from glutamic acid and cysteine. Glutamine-cysteine is synthesized with glycocol to give rise to a tripeptide called glutathione. Both reactions require the presence of ATP and Mg and in the second stage.

Condensation of glycol with benzoic acid, which is toxic to the body, forms hippuric acid, a non-toxic substance: Threonine is a gluco-forming amino acid that starts its biosynthesis from aspartic acid with the consumption of 2ATP and the participation of NADP. In the carboxylation stage of leucine, hydroxymethyl-glutamine CoA is formed, an important compound in protein metabolism. The activation reaction is a complex endergonic

process that requires the presence of activated CO_2 and is performed in the presence of a biotin enzyme and ATP as an energy donor. In transmethylation processes, methionine activation is an enzymatic process that requires the presence of Mg and reduced glutathione. The reaction takes place in the presence of ATP which, by dissolving three molecules of phosphoric acid, releases the adenosyl radical which binds to the sulfur atom in the methionine molecule:

methionine + ATP ------> CH_3 - S - adenosylmethionine + H_3PO_4

The energy of the macro-ergic phosphate bonds in ATP is transferred to the methyl bile group. Upon activation, methionine in the form of adenosine methionine participates in a series of transmethylation reactions on specific acceptors (norepinephrine --> adrenaline). The biosynthesis of coenzymes with nucleotide structure, in which the participation of nucleotides is necessary, is done with the help of nucleotide triphosphates, especially with the participation of ATP.

A category of coenzymes comes from vitamins, especially from the B group of vitamins. Thus, riboflavin (vitamin B2) can be phosphorylated to form flavin-nucleotide (FMN) or riboflavin monophosphate.

Riboflavin -- ATP --> FMN + ADP

FMN can react with another molecule of ATP to form FAD-ul (flavin-adenine-nucleotide): FMN + ATP ------> FAD + PP2. The structure of NAD and NADP is also a nucleotide structure. Coenzyme A also has a partially nucleotide structure and its biosynthesis requires the participation of ATP. The structure of vitamin B12 also recognizes a fragment with a nucleotide structure consisting of dimethyl-benzidine-imidazole, pentose, phosphoric acid. ATP is also involved in activating other vitamins to convert them to coenzymes or enzymes. This is the case with thiamine, pyridoxal, biotin, lipoic acid. The reactions are as follows:

Thiamine + ATP -> Thiamine-PPi, (Pyridoxal), + AMP
Pyridoxal + ATP --> Pyridoxal-P + Biotin + ATP-->Biotin-adenine + PPi
Biotin-adenine + enzyme --> Biotin-enzyme + AMP
Lipoate + ATP - -> Lipoate-adenylate + PPi

It has been found that enzymes called DNA polymerases (I, II, III) and ligases are involved in DNA biosynthesis. DNA polymerase I is mainly involved in the repair of modified DNA under the influence of various factors. The main features of the process are:

a). the corresponding nucleoside triphosphates, mono and inactive diphosphates are involved in the reactions, which means that a high energy is required to carry out this process;

b). in order for the reaction to take place, the presence of all four nucleotide triphosphates (ATP, GTP, CTP, TTP) is required; the absence of one of them implies polycondensation

c). the reaction depends on the presence of Mg + ions;

d). a preformed DNA is required to carry out the reaction;

e). The DNA-RNA system reaction also has a nucleophilic mechanism by which the nucleophilic 3-OH group binds to the phosphoryl group in the nucleotide triphosphate releasing pyrophosphate. DNA ligases complement the action of polymerases allowing the creation of 3'-5 'diester bonds on which the formation of a circular molecular bond is initiated.

The action of DNA ligases requires the participation of ATP as well as other factors: - in tumor cells the transcription has from RNA-DNA-RNA under the action of reverse polymerase DNA polymerase-transcriptase;

- DNA biosynthesis could be determined by highlighting 9x104 intra-nucleotide bonds per minute. Frequently the cell can "repair" the altered nucleic acid under the action of endonucleases. Through these enzymes the modified fragment is removed from the nucleic acid molecule, and under the action of DNA polymerases a direct nucleotide fragment is introduced, the process being controlled by the pre-existing matrix DNA in the cell.

Changes in the structure of DNA, the carrier of genetic information, can occur in larger portions, leading to changes in the structure of the reproductive process. At the same time, ATP is an activator of allosteric enzymes. In some enzymes, enzymatic phosphorylation results in their activation or inactivation. Glutamine synthetase consists of 12 units that modify their activity by introducing a residue of AMP from ATP into each of the 12 subunits and thus inactivates. In the case of glutamine synthetase, the activation of the enzyme takes place through a process of phosphorylase.

Transferases are a class of enzymes that catalyze a reaction such as: R - A + R '- B ----------> R - B' + R '- A wherein part of the molecule of a substrate called a donor is transferred to another layer called an acceptor:

a). Trans-methylases are a class of enzymes that transfer the methyl group from the donor to the acceptor according to the reaction: R - CH3 + R '- H ---> R - H + R' - CH3 ⇓.

The transformation of the apparent donor substrate into the actual donor substrate is done by oxidation reaction or by charging with energy released by ATP. Example: ATP + methionine ---> S - adenosylmethionine ⇓ -+ H3PO4

b). trans-acetylase transfers acyl groups (acyl residues) from donors to receptors. Activation of organic acids by their transformation into acyl-CoA derivatives is done by providing ATP. The overall acetic acid activation reaction can be formulated as follows:

CH3 - COOH + CoA: SH + ATP ----> CH3 - CO ~ S - CoA + AMP + PPi Acetic acid ⇓ ---- CoA acid.

The reactions are catalyzed by specific enzymes in the liver and other tissues. Nucleotide phosphorylases catalyze the transfer reaction of the residue of ribose 1-phosphate from ribose 1,5-bisphosphate to adenine, with nucleotide formation: **ribose - 1.5 diphosphate + adenine -------> AMP + H3PO4 ⇓ Phosphokinases catalyze the general reaction: ATP + X ---> ADP + X-P**

These enzymes play an important role in biosynthetic processes because they allow the release of energy accumulated in the macro-energetic phosphate bonds in the ATP molecule. Among the most important phosphokinases are:

a) hexokinase b) phosphokinases;

c) tri-phospho-glycero-kinases; d) pyruvate kinase; e) myokinase; f) creatine kinase; g) nucleotide diphospho-kinases. Nucleotide di-phosphokinase catalyzes the transfer of phosphate from ATP to UDP (uridindin-phosphate) or IDP (inosinidin-phosphate) after reactions:

UDP + ATP --> UTP + ADP IDP + ATP -> ITP + ADP

Biotin plays an important role in carboxylation-decarboxylation reactions. Decarboxylation enzymes require the presence of ATP for their activity: ATP + biotin enzyme --> ADP biotin enzyme + H_3PO_4 This complex reacts with CO_2 which, by substituting ADP, forms a new CO_2 complex - the biotin enzyme.

This pasture elates the macro-energic bond and represents an activated CO_2 capable of participating in carboxylation reactions: ADP - biotin enzyme + CO_2 -> CO_2 – biotin-enzyme + ADP Ligases, known as synthetases, catalyze the formation of a bond between two molecules in the presence of ATP as an energy donor.

X + Y + ATP --> X - Y + ATP + PPi ⇓, (reversible reaction)

Among the most important ligases are carboxylases that act on the type reaction:

R - H + CO_2 + H_2O + ATP --> R - COOH + ADP + Pi ⇓.

DNA topoisomerase, recently discovered as a malignancy factor, is 20 times higher in cancer cells than in normal cells. This enzyme helps in the transcription of malignant DNA in very large quantities. Research continues. Biotin is a B-complex vitamin and acts as a coenzyme, a carrier of CO_2 during the carboxylation process that can be released in biosynthesis processes on an acceptor pyruvate:

Acetic acid + CO_2 + ATP + H_2O --> oxalyl-acetic acid carboxylase

The energy resulting from the degradation of large biomolecules to small molecules can be used at least partially in biosynthetic processes after its prior storage in compounds containing macro-ergic bonds.

Through their hydrolysis, the biochemical energy necessary for the biosynthesis of various natural organic compounds is formed, as they are consumed, formed and then regenerated during metabolic processes, thus fulfilling the role of coenzymes in addition to enzymes called kinases. Coenzyme A consists of a phosphorylated ATP residue, a pantothenic acid residue and a cysteine residue.

Its function is based on the ability of the SH group of cysteamine to bind through macro-energic thioester bonds, acyl radicals in general, and especially acetyl radicals, which can be transferred during metabolism to appropriate receptors. Thiamine pyrophosphate is derived from the

phosphorylation of thiamine with ATP and is the coenzyme of the processes of decarboxylation of aceto-acids, trans-acetylation, phospho-acetylation. pyruvate decarboxylase Pyruvic acid --> acetic aldehyde then PP From the above we can conclude that ATP performs a transfer of functional groups. It contains two macro-energic bonds, the hydrolysis of which results in the energy required for endergonic biosynthetic processes.

Phosphate groups in the ATP molecule can be cleaved gradually or completely, by hydrolysis of ATP to result in ADP, AMP, adenosine and phosphate (Pi) or pyrophosphate (PPi) ions. ATP resynthesis takes place due to the energy resulting from tissue respiration, aerobic degradation of glucose, oxidation of fatty acids, etc. The cleavage of ATP into ADP + Pi is done by ATPase, and the released energy is usually used to activate a substrate to be activated. Following the interaction of ATP with GDP, GTP and ADP will form, under the action of a guanyl-cyclase from GTP, cGMP can form, which, like cAMP, acts as a mediator of the action of certain categories of hormones. From the set of ATP converted to cAMP by an adenyl cyclase with cGMP will give rise to a permanent cellular bioenergetic reflux that underlies cell life.

Major energy source of the cell is the oxidation of the substrates of food principles in O2 from the air, transported by blood to the tissues. The living cell obtains its energy by oxidizing the hydrogen released from the organic substrate processed by the body, the formation of CO2 appearing as a secondary phenomenon, often dependent only indirectly on oxidation reactions, which ultimately lead to decarboxylation. Numerous unknowns and many uncertainties over the years of medical research have made it almost impossible to delineate the preclinical phase of a chronic disease from the initial state of health. The detection of biochemical changes in the body's apparatus and systems prior to their clinical expression has been quite uncertain through investigations conducted with the usual paraclinical means, [3].

CHAPTER IV

BIOENERGETICS OF THE NORMAL CELL

The energy apparatus of the cell is represented by the set of mitochondria. Mitochondrial infrastructures are represented by the outer membrane, the intermembrane space, the inner membrane, the mitochondrial crystals and the mitochondrial matrix. As can be seen in the diagram below, the mitochondrial membranes are separated from each other by a usually optically empty, homogeneous space, called the peri-mitochondrial space of about 100 A arranged perpendicular to the major axis of the mitochondria. Using special techniques, it was possible to locate on the inner mitochondrial membrane some small, spherical particles, fixed to this wall either through the pedicle or directly.

Called oxy-some, these particles play an important role in the transfer of the inside of the mitochondria. Mitochondria selectively accumulate mineral ions (K^{+}, Na^{+}, Mg^{2+} and Ca^{2+}), vitamins (A, C, B2, B6, B12, E) and numerous enzymes. Some of them cause the phenomenon of acetylation (acetyl CoA, acyltransferase), others enter the mitochondrial respiratory chain, (cytochromes), the Krebs cycle (dehydrogenases), and others catalyze the oxidation of fatty acids, initiate gluconeogenesis or couple oxidation with phosphorylation").

The chemical analysis also showed that in the membranes there are water-insoluble enzymes and in the matrix water-soluble enzymes and the mentioned metal ions, RNA, DNA, and nucleotides all deriving from adenine such as APM, ADP, ATP (as well as coenzymes NAD, NADP), which would constitute all the phosphorous, non-lipid compounds of mitochondria.

The following biochemical processes take place in the mitochondria:

- porphyrin biosynthesis (basal nuclei of cytochromes);
- redox-active protein biosynthesis;
- biosynthesis of mitochondrial structural proteins through mitochondrial ribosomes;
- "de novo" biosynthesis of amino acids;

- polymerization of own nucleic acids;
- partial manufacture of the nucleotides needed to catalyze the flow of electron transfer.

The final stage of ADP phosphorylation --> ATP is attributed exclusively to the terminal spheres of repetitive mutations in the inner membrane, and the process of respiratory electron transfer is located in their based parts. The contacted condensed form of mitochondria will correspond to its active respiration in the presence of ATP, and the ballooned form represents the state of anaerobiosis lacking ATP. Mitochondrial respiration depends on the concentration of ATP and the substrate to be oxidized, there is a control of this by balancing the terminal reaction of phosphorylation ATP --> ADP + Pi, <-- both through the dehydrogenation steps of the Krebs cycle.

The possibility of using ADP + Pi in ATP synthesis is related to the presence of respiratory substrates (succinate, pyruvate, etc.). The ATP molecule, considered the universal carrier of secured energy, due to its ability to mobilize the terminal phosphoric group, generates ADP, with energy release, while creating a reserve of unsaturated nucleotide, necessary for O2 consumption in the presence of the substrate. Green et al. (1963) concluded that research on animal mitochondria concluded that there was an impressive quantity of macromolecular units in mitochondrial membranes, each of which could transfer electrons from succinate and NADH to the Krebs cycle. to molecular oxygen. They named these particles ETP (electron-transport-protein). In the mitochondria, a soluble protein factor F1 "was isolated which catalyzes the synthesis" of ATP during oxidation by intervening in the transformation of X - P1 + ADP --> ATP. This type of reaction forms 1.8 moles of ATP formed for one mole of O2 consumed. Ca2 + and phosphate supplementation of coupled mitochondria results in a net stimulation of respiration with the parallel accumulation of Ca and P in the matrix space. As the levels of Ca2 + and P decrease, the respiratory stages of the isolated mitochondria undergo a transition to anoxemia. ATP synthesis depends on the concentration of H + or OH ions ", and the meaning of reactions would take place according to the formula:

ATP + H2O + 2H + -> ADP + Pi + 2H + Mitochondrial interior

-- Mitochondrial exterior hence the protons are released to the outside of the inner membrane. In this way, ATP synthesis occurs as a result of the concentrations of electrical charges on the surface of the mitochondrial membrane which causes an increased H + potential increased on the outside and is reduced on the inside by the formation of water. It has been observed

that exogenous cytoplasmic, glycolytic ATP produces the distension of coupled mitochondria and endogenous intramitochondrial ATP in high concentrations causes agglomeration of native mitochondrial suspensions, **[Figure 2].**

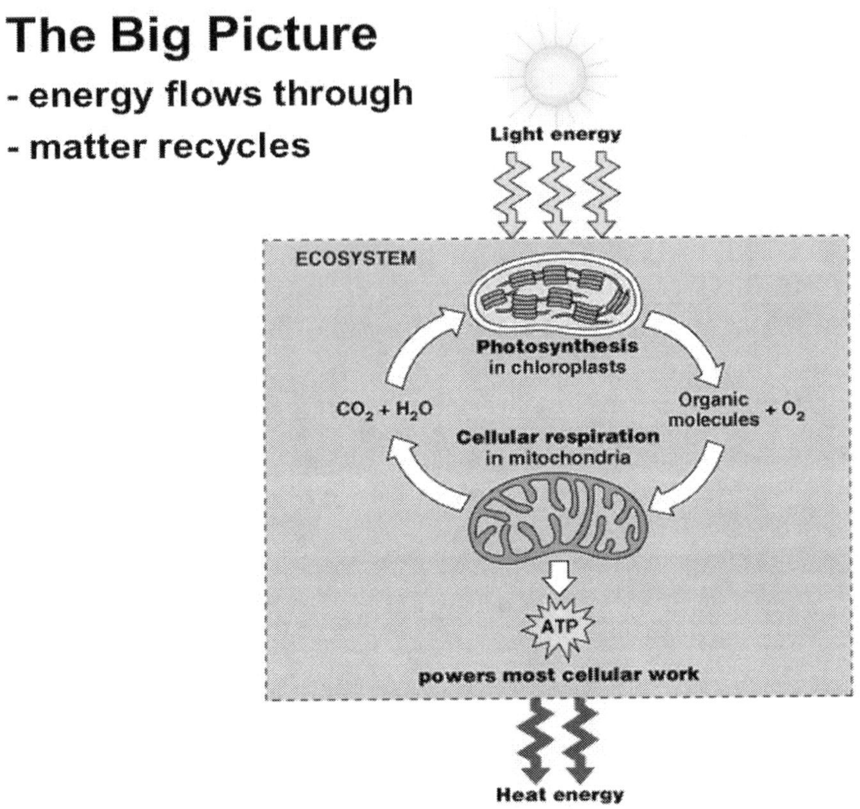

Figure 2: ATP synthesis in plants by photosynthesis process

Particular matrix cationic proteins in the mitochondria can inhibit the molecular functions of ATP at certain stoichiometric concentrations. This process of inhibiting ATP functions is stopped by alkaline pH values. Ongoing research has shown that the meaning of synthesis reactions ADP + Pi --> ATP + H2O can be reproducibly controlled in vitro, depending on the concentration of system factors, pH and ionic strength appearing likely to exist a functional control of energy by creating weak bonds between chemical complexes of newly formed biologically active substances.

Chronic tissue diseases under the action of an infectious factor are sustained by changes in tissue pH, tissue electrical potential, and created energy deficit (A. Pischinger et al., 1991). Infection or trauma causes acidosis in the affected tissue segment, causing tissue shock, increased Mg + and decreased Ca in the blood, followed in a few days by counter shock (under conditions of a normal defence capacity) the symptoms of the infection becoming clinically visible. Finally, there are minor variations of the mineral substances, corresponding to the convalescence phase.

This reaction is regulated by the fundamental system, including the humoral one. The intensity of the energy reaction depends on the intensity of the installed acidosis. The greater the energy difference between the initial stage and the reaction to infection or trauma, the greater the amount of energy released. In long-lasting acidosis, the difference between the initial pH value and that during an infection decreases, and the energy released may not be enough to trigger the defence processes.

Most likely there is an energy deficit. Through the continuous process of repolarization and depolarization of the cell membrane under the action of toxic factors, a lot of energy is consumed, in infectious foci and ATP deficiency, in addition to the biophysical effects due to the focus, being inhibited and biochemical functions. Mitochondrial ATP deficiency is 18% in systemic inflammatory diseases, 30-34% in malignant tumors (normal value is 107-148 m V / ml / 10 minutes).

L8 107 = 2.02 µM / ATP L8 107 = 2.17 µM / ATP Energy Deficiency in Triggering Defensive

Reactions in Fundamental Tissue Also Delays Immune Response. Returning strictly to the mitochondria, it seems that the surface of the inner membrane is directly related to the respiratory intensity of the tissue. Some electron transporters are organized into supramolecular complexes that can be isolated from the membrane. Such a complex contains NADH-dehydrogenase, 4 or more iron-sulfur centres and many lipids.

Cytochromes a and a3 form another complex. These "respiratory" assemblies are located in the inner membrane at regular intervals. Some metabolites such as nucleotides, di- and tri-carboxylic acids, fatty acids, amino acids, and various cations cannot enter and exit freely through the inner membrane of the mitochondria.

Their transport is done selectively, with the help of specific carriers that have three distinct features:

• specific transporters have saturation kinetics just like the saturation of substrate enzymes;

• carriers are specific to a substrate or group of substrates;

• Carriers may be specifically inhibited without affecting other carriers.

The inner membrane of the mitochondria is also impermeable to NADH, H +. If dehydrogenation of the substrate has occurred in the cytoplasm, it is necessary to transfer H to the mitochondria through a transporter capable of crossing the membrane.

Enzymes called mitochondrial flavin-dehydrogenases to take up hydrogen from mitochondrial NADH as well as from flavin enzymes and transfer it to another component of the respiratory chain, ubiquinone.

Some mitochondrial flavin enzymes contain non-hemin iron which is bound to the - SH group of cysteine residues in the protein. It is likely that this iron, like that of cytochromes, functions as an intermedius. Electron transporter flavoprotein (FTF) is involved in accepting electrons from mitochondrial FADH2 which is unable to transmit it directly to ubiquitn, UQ, (or coenzyme Q) which is a component of the mitochondrial respiratory chain electron acceptor oscillating between the reduced and oxidized form.

Its participation in the respiratory chain is based on its property of forming a redox system. The submitochondrial particles of the inner membrane can be fragmented into four complexes:

a).• Complex I contains flavoproteins (FP) that cause oxidation of NADH, H + reducing UQ.

•b). Complex H has a similar role, but in the oxidation of succinate:

c). Orderly assembly of these complexes in the inner membrane of go-to insurance to ensure cellular bioenergy as long as they remain intact and are not inhibited by specific inhibitors while allowing the cyclic crossing of the oxalacetic acid (oxalacetate) initiator of the Krebs cycle in combination with Acetyl CoA (pyruvate derivative), the common intermediate of degradation of food principles: carbohydrates, lipids, proteins.

Because the generation of ATP by exogenous biological oxidation reactions can be considered a primary function of mitochondria, the mitochondrial ADP transporter and ATP outside the mitochondria are of great importance.

The two adenyl nucleotides move simultaneously but in reverse: ADP enters the mitochondria and ATP exits the mitochondria. The transport involved in this process is strictly specific for these two nucleotides and the exchange always takes place.

As a result, the ADP + ATP pole in the mitochondria is maintained at a constant level. Because the exchange of ADP / ATP is in the form of anions, given that ATP has a higher negative charge than ADP, the exchange of the two anions takes place with an energy consumption of approx. 3 Kcal.

Another indispensable factor for bioenergy: mitochondria is calcium. Ca^{2+} accumulation in the mitochondria occurs through "active" transport that is energy dependent. In the absence of O_2 or oxidizable substrates, Ca^{2+} transport to the mitochondria can only be done if ATP is added. The apparent decoupling effect of adding Ca^{2+} to a mitochondrial suspension is more accurately explained by diverting some of the energy that is commonly used for ATP synthesis to be used to accumulate Ca^{2+} in the mitochondria.

These two processes are energy accepting systems and alternatives in mitochondria. Substrate > 2e ---> O_2 or ADP + H_2PO_4 ATP cation accumulation.

Other cations, such as Na^+ K^+ are also actively transported but the physiological significance of this transport is lower compared to that of Ca^{2+}. Maintaining the components of the respiratory chain in a correct spatial position in the mitochondrial membrane is likely to be accomplished by a "structural protein" that acts as a cian-hydrophobic. Determining the degree of oxidation of the various components of the respiratory chain, spectrophotometrically, on the intact mitochondria, showed that the mitochondria work in a "stationary state" regime. It constantly receives substrates in the cytoplasm, which it transforms into final products.

The respiratory chain works under optical conditions as a continuous production line. Each stage of the process operates at a constant rate, the molecules of each carrier are alternately reduced and oxidized so that the flow of electrons is permanently ensured. The process is dynamic so that the proportion of oxidized and reduced forms is constant at all times. At the initial end of the chain, its components are predominantly in the reduced form, and at the terminal end in the oxidized form. ATP is the energy "currency" of the cell.

For each oxygen atom consumed by the respiratory chain H3PO4 ester 3 molecules of ATP are formed, the ratio = 3 in case of oxidation nO2 concentration. NAD substrates - dependent. If the oxidation of the substrate is done by FAD, such as succinate, only two molecules of ATP result, the ratio P: O = 2. The location of the three phosphorylation points in the respiratory chain are complexes I, III and IV.

This location coincides with the highest unevenness of the redox potential and therefore with the places where the greatest amount of energy is released. In intact mitochondria, respiration cannot occur without concomitant phosphorylation of ADP to ATP. The availability of ADP, substrate and oxygen are three of the most important factors controlling the rate of respiration. Under certain conditions, the level of inorganic phosphate and ATP can also affect the rate of functioning of the respiratory chain. Oz consumed with ADP.

The ratio is the best respiratory control index O2 consumed without ADP. In intact mitochondria, it has a value between 5 -20, while in decoupled mitochondria the respiratory index is equal to 1. ADP + H3PO4 ---> ATP This is consumed. It's preserved In the inner membrane of the mitochondria is an ATPase that catalyzes ATP hydrolysis:

ATP + H2O --------> H3PO4 + ADP

Although this reaction is inverse to that of ATP formation, the enzyme is of great interest because it is activated by DNF and is likely to participate in at least one of the steps of phosphorylating ADP to ATP.

ATPase works reversibly, being one of the decoupling factors on the inner surface of the inner mitochondrial membrane. Earlier we mentioned that the outer membrane is practically permeable to all metabolites, while the inner mitochondrial membrane is generally impermeable, the transport of metabolites being done selectively. The inner membrane of the mitochondria can allow acids to penetrate without being actively transported. This category includes the basic fuels of mitochondrial oxidation: pyruvate, fatty acids and ketone bodies. These monocarboxylic acids enter the mitochondria in an undissociated form.

R-COO + H + ---> R-COOH --R - COOH ---> R- COO + H

The di- and tri-carboxylic acids of the Krebs cycle are transported to the mitochondria in the form of anions, and to maintain electroneutrality during passage through the inner membrane, an anion with a similar charge must

leave the mitochondria at the same time. Phosphoric acid is transported to the mitochondria in an undissociated form.

This independent transport makes the phosphate available for exchange with malic or succinic acid, components of the Krebs cycle. Fumaric and oxal-acetic acids are unable to penetrate the membrane. Citric acid, isocitrate and ketoglutarate are also transported to the mitochondria in the form of anions, but their transport is done by exchange with malic acid and not phosphate. The inner membrane is impermeable to NAD +, NADH, CoA and acyl CoA. As these substances exist in both the matrix and the cytoplasm, the barrier formed by the inner membrane separates them into two poles, intramitochondrial and extra-mitochondrial.

The changes between the two compartments, however, occur in both directions. It is known, for example, that during glycolysis NADH is formed in the cytoplasm, resulting in the oxidation of phospho-glyceraldehyde. H-transport of NADH from the cytoplasm to the mitochondria is accomplished by a "shuttle mechanism" of irreversibly acting dihydroxyacetone phosphate and glycerol-P and reversibly acting malate-oxaloacetate.

We believe that the electron goes from NADH to O2 through an exergonic process.

NADH + 1/2 O2 + H --> H2O + NAD + ß -ΔG = - 526 kcal / mol, (reversible reaction)

Free oxidation energy is used in ATP synthesis:

Mitochondrial ATPase (H +) ADP + Pi + H -> ATP + H2O ß, (reversible reaction)

PH gradient and membrane potential! is the driving force of the proton that is used in ATP synthesis. The H + concentration becomes high at the mitochondrial cytosolic site and an electric potential is created in this place. This proton, "motive force" of 0.224 V corresponds to free energy of 5.2 Kcal per proton molecule. Δ Go for the electronic transfer from NADH to the lower energy with NADH-Q reductase and is -12 Kcal/mol.

Cytochrome „b" to C1 = - 1Occal / mol;
- From cytochrome "a" to O2 = -24kcal / mol.

The transfer of the electron through each of the energy storage sites transmits conformational changes with the ejection of the proton from the

matrix to the cytoplasmic site. In the reaction: ADP3- + P2 + H2 --> ATP + H2O. the terminal oxygen in ADP attracts the P2 atom to form a Penta-covalent intermediate bond which then dissociates into ATP + H2O. This reaction requires the participation of Mg 2+ accompanied by ATP synthetase, known as H + - ATPase or FoF1 - ATPase, where: Fo = conducting proton, F1 = synthesized ATP. This database consists of pol-peptide chains with 3B3Y stoichiometry:

The attraction of O2 to ADP and the distribution of O2 to Pi occupy the top of a triangular pyramid. The energizing proton passing through Fo produces the catalysis of Fo / F1 and O2 goes to Pi changing the balance towards ATP synthesis. The positive membrane potential causes a high concentration of H + at the junction of FoF1 - ATP-synthetase subunits. The mitochondrial ring membrane is impermeable to NADH and NAD +, **{Scheme 4|**.

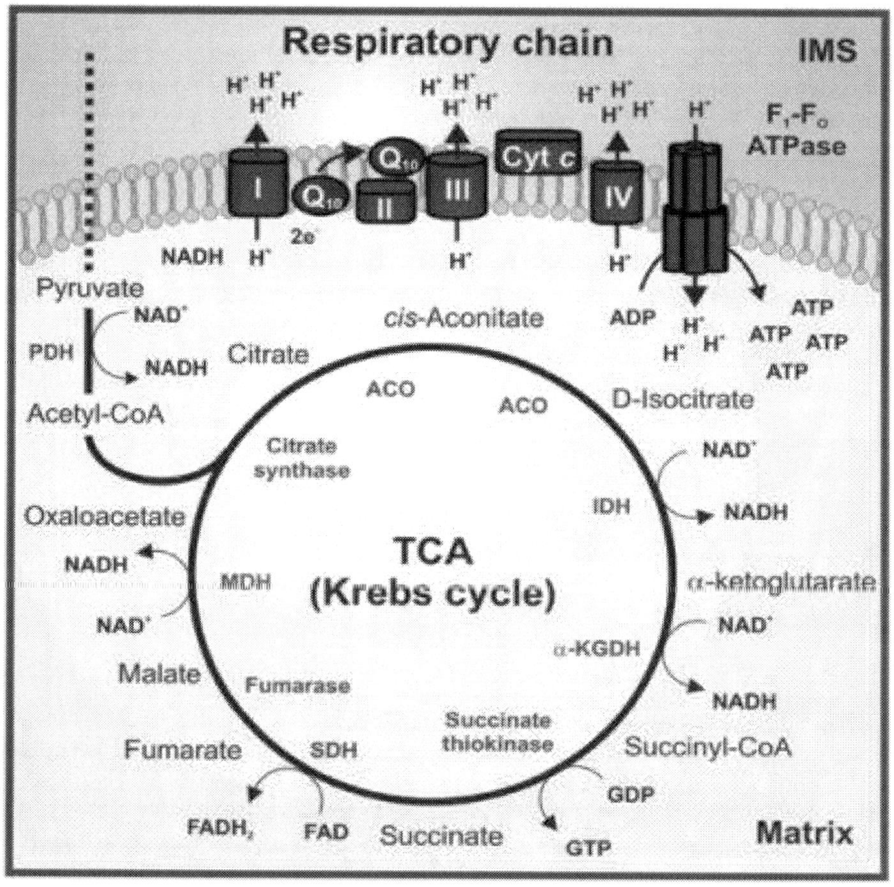

Scheme 4. *Vital functions of mitochondria with respiratory chine*

Respiratory complexes actively extrude protons from the mitochondrial matrix, thereby generating an electrochemical gradient that is dissipated by the -ATP synthase to generate ATP. The TCA cycle (also known as the Krebs cycle) is the an-other bioenergetic pathway that is virtually confined to the mitochondrial matrix. In normal conditions, the end-product of glycolysis (pyruvate) is taken up by mitochondria, promptly converted to acetyl-CoA and CO by the PDH complex, and feeds into the TCA cycle.

Through the TCA, acetyl-CoA is fully oxidized to CO, whereas three NADH, one FADH and one GTP (or ATP) molecules are generated. Of note, the reducing equivalents provided by NADH and FADH can be used

by respiratory complexes to produce the ATPase part of oxidative phosphorylation. Mitochondria provided an optimal biochemical microenvironment for (at least part of) several other biochemical cascades, including the urea cycle, gluconeogenesis, and ketogenesis;

But NADH is formed by glycolysis in the cytoplasm by oxidation of glyceraldehyde-3-phosphate and NAD + must be regenerated by continuous glycolysis. How cytoplasmic NADH can then oxidize the respiratory chain The solution is that electrons from NADH, other than NADH itself, have been brought over the outer mitochondrial membrane. For the first time in this process, the electron is transferred from NADH to dihydroxyacetone.

The reaction is catalyzed by 3-phosphate dehydrogenase which occurs in the cytosol. This energy process is predominant in muscles where there is an increase in oxidative phosphorylation. In the liver and heart, the cytoplasmic NADP electron is brought to the mitochondria by the malate-aspartate pathway. NADH --> NAD + -> NAD + + NADH mitochondrial cytoplasmic mitochondrial cytoplasmic).

By transferring NADH, 3 molecules of ATP are synthesized with transferred NADH. The entry of ADP into the mitochondria is coupled with the exit of ATP, by ATP - ADP - translocase a specific transporter protein called adenine carrier. ADP enters the mitochondrial matrix only if ATP exits and vice versa. The translocase catalyzed reaction is: **ADPc3- + ATPm4- -> ADPm3- + ATPc4** in which the subscription "c" denotes the cytosolic site and "m" is the matrix site in the mitochondrial ring.

Translocase is a dimer consisting of 30 subunits. ATP is transferred out of the cell 30 "earlier than ADP and ATP has a higher negative charge. The membrane potential decreases by changing ATP to ADP, resulting in a net transfer of negative charge out of the matrix. The transfer of electrons through the respiratory chain regenerates the membrane potential consumed by this process.

Electrons do not usually pass through the respiratory chain until ADP is phosphorylated to ATP. Oxidative phosphorylation permanently requires NADH, or another higher-potential electron source, O2, ADP, and Pi. The most important factor in determining the rate of oxidative phosphorylation is the level of ADP. The rate of O2 consumed by homogeneous tissues increases markedly when ADP is added and returns to baseline when ADP has been converted to ATP. ATP levels affect the rate of citric acid because

it needs NAD + and FAD +. ADP levels increase when ATP is consumed, so oxidative phosphorylation is coupled with ATP.

Electrons do not pass through the molecule chain to O2 unless ATP needs to be synthesized. Here is another model for regulating energy exchange. This justifies the role of active physical movement in maintaining a high rate of electron flow at the mitochondrial level. Dinitrophenol (DNF) and other aromatic acids decrease the chemical energy of mitochondrial intermembrane and decrease ATP production. ATP is synthesized when the proton returns to the mitochondrial matrix through an enzyme complex.

The ATP turnaround is very high. For example, a person consumes 4 kg of ATP at rest in 24 hours. During stress, and exercise, the use of ATP can be higher than 0.5 kg/min. Regarding bioenergetic changes, the electrostatic repulsion between the negative charge groups is reduced when ATP is hydrolyzed, when the energy of the phosphoric molecule becomes lower. Another factor in the elimination of bioenergy from ATP is that the potential in ATP is high and ADP + Pi enjoys a high stabilizing resonance against ATP.

A thermodynamically un-favorable reaction can be converted to a favorable one by coupling it with a sufficient number of molecules. Hydrolysis of "n" molecules of ATP changes the balance of the reaction sequences by a factor of 10. **A + ATP + H2O --> B + ADP - Pi + H + ß, (reversible reaction)**

In transformation, A -> B is consumed (+) 4 kcal but the free energy of the reaction becomes ΔGo == -3.3 kcal. A and B may show conformational differences in proteins. ATP synthesized by oxidative phosphorylation is a source of aerobic ATP in the body. Alternatively, the electron-derived potential can be used for biosynthesis which reduces ATP levels. Metabolic reactions are controlled and go through the energy status of the cell. An indicator of energy status is the energy load:

ATP +1/2 ADP : Se=------------------------- ATP + ADP + AMP

The cellular energy load can have a value from O > 1. Daniel Atkinson showed that ATP generated in one way is inhibited by another energy load if using ATP in another way stimulates another energy load for which it is not intended. Thus, the energy charge, like the pH in the cells, is buffered. In muscle cells, it was observed that after 20 'of exercise the level of PC decreased markedly while the orthophosphate increased markedly.

In contrast, ATP levels remained almost constant. In physical exertion, after 6-12 ', by installing aerobic status, pyruvate enters the mitochondria where it is completely oxidized to CO_2 and H_2O.

If the O_2 ratio becomes insufficient, pyruvate no longer enters the Krebs cycle and is converted to lactate. The central enzyme of glycolysis remains phosphofructokinase which is allosterically controlled by ATP. We also remind you that the level of phosphofructokinase is inhibited by the high level of ATP which decreases its affinity for F-6-P.

Citrate formed in the Krebs cycle, slightly crossing the mitochondrial membranes will inhibit phosphofructokinase. Fatty acids formed in the cytoplasm either by the hydrolysis of fats or by biosynthesis are oxidized intra-mitochondrially. For this, the fatty acids are inactivated for the action of acyl-CoA synthetase to Acetyl-CoA with the participation of ATP from which AMP + PPi will arise. Since the mitochondrial membrane is impermeable to RCO-SCoA acyl derivatives, they are converted under the action of carnitine acyl transferase to acylcarnitine, which passes easily through the mitochondrial membrane.

On the inner side of the mitochondrial membrane, acyl-carnitine derivatives are transformed into carnitine and the Acyl-CoA molecule, which are oxidized in the process of β oxidation. The limiting step in the regulation of fatty acid oxidation in mitochondria is the activity of carnitine-acyl transferase, especially intramitochondrial activity which controls the amount of acyl-CoA that can enter the β oxidation process.

Recall that in the immediate energy needs, pyruvic acid will initially enter the mitochondria and will be oxidatively decarboxylated to acetyl-CoA, and this will combine with oxaloacetate imitating the Krebs cycle, of varying intensity imposed by metabolic conversions at some point. Bear citrate can cross the mitochondrial membrane and enter the cytoplasm, where it will break down into acetyl-CoA which will synthesize fatty acids and oxaloacetate which, passing into malate and then pyruvate, will re-enter the Krebs cycle.

This citric acid circuit has been dubbed the "reserve withdrawal" and takes place with the participation of NAD-NADH and NADP-NADPH. Referring to some cells in the blood system, we make the first mention that the energy source for the maturation of the erythrocytes is a glycolytic reaction left on a scale involved, in the conversion of glucose into lactic acid by which the ATP concentration is maintained. ATP in erythrocytes has several functions:

- is used to absorb plasma glucose;
- maintains the level of intracellular K and extracellular Na;
- maintains the biconcave shape of the red blood cell;
- participates in cell synthesis and metabolism;
- keeps Hb low.

The absence of these properties is observed in ATP-deficient cells, as a result of prolonged storage "in vitro" or as a consequence of incubation in the absence of an energy source (substrate). However, Centro-cystic glycolytic activity maintains ATP levels above 1.4 μM ml of cells by phosphorylating ADP during the conversion of glucose to lactic acid. In platelets, ATP ensures their proper functioning and effectively participates in platelet aggregation.

The human lymphocyte is low in glycogen and has an aerobic and anaerobic metabolic pathway. Hexose-monophosphate is present but is metabolized by less than 1%. At rest, lymphocytes consume more O2 than granulocytes, mainly through glycolysis and Krebs acid. Inhibition of glycolysis by O2 (Pasteur effect) can be demonstrated in lymphocytes, a demonstration that will lead to cellular respiratory inhibition with the accumulation of glucose in high concentrations. Na-K-dependent ATPase activity is 3-fold higher in lymphocyte cells than in granulocyte cells. A decrease in leukocyte glycogen levels was measured in patients with LGC compared to normal, while an increase in glycogen levels was found in patients with myeloid metaplasia, polycythemia vera, and leukocytosis.

Busulfan treatment normalizes glycogen levels. High levels of NAD were found in ALL and LGC and we found high levels of ATP in CLL lymphocytes. Glycogen is low in LGC leukocytes but is high in agranulocytosis. In normal subjects, granulocytes are the first exception to the theory presented above. Granulocyte cellular ATP is much more sensitive to the inhibition of glycolysis than to the inhibition of respiration.

In LGC, glycolysis decreases very little in the presence of O2, which suggests that the Pasteur effect is not fully operative in these cells. Warburg observed that the effect of Pasteur, the inhibition of glycolysis under aerobic conditions, was greatly diminished in tissue tumors, and formulated the idea that the absence of the Pasteur effect is a feature of malignant tumor cells. In this paper, for the determination of cellular bioenergy, we did not measure the intensity of the phenomenon as such, expressed in the apparatus and systems of the body in the form of the biofield, but we relied on the

existence of this phenomenon in the generation of cellular ATP. acting as an energy storage molecule.

The works of S. Kirlian, Szent-Gyorgy, V. Adamenco, W. Sedlak, and Eugen Celan demonstrated the presence of energy configurations that accompany them. The physical structure of biological organisms and which many authors bring together under the name of bioplasm. The process of electron transfer is seen by some researchers as a physical process, while others consider it electrochemical,

responsible for the production of electroluminescence. However, in a reduced schematization it can be seen as:

$A\text{-}A^{+} + e\ A +$,,,,,,,,,,,, $A * A + hv$

$A\text{-}\ A^{-} + e\ A^{-}$;;;;;;;;;;;;;; $A * A + hv$

A = molecule of the luminescent substance; A + and A- = cationic and anionic radicals. The assumptions of most knowledgeable researchers of the problem converge on the idea of the existence of an energy structure organized in the volume of the biological organism which exceeds its anatomical barrier. The peri-proximal area of this energetic structure, which can be highlighted by electrographic processes, delimits the so-called "aura".

Russian and Polish and Polish authors, who support the bio-plasmatic field, are inclined to consider this energy field as a definite presence, responsible for the production of a whole series of phenomena based on its perimeter. The phenomenon of super-based bioluminescence began to be investigated in 1955, thanks to the work of L. Colin, V. Facchini and A. Rossi. Later, beginning in 1961, he was studied by B.N. Tarusov, T.G. Mamedov, et al., And since 1976 by F.A. Popp, W. Nagl, B. Ruth, et al. The current general opinion is almost unanimous in considering that super-low-grade bioluminescence is characteristic of the entire living biological world. The phenomenon is characterized by a variable photonic emission, whose intensity covers very wide limits, ranging from 103 quanta/sec recorded in pea root growth areas and up to 15 - 50n photons/sec and cm^2. of the biomass surface recorded in bacteria, fungi, insects, some plant and animal tissues.

In humans, the level recorded for liver and bone marrow cells was determined in the range of 200 - 2000 photons/sec and cm^2. biomass surface area. The general appearance of the emission curve of the super-faint luminescence seems to be identical for most organisms, which makes some

authors hypothesize the possible possibility of quasi-identical mechanisms for its production, the differences being mainly related to the kinetics of the process. Each person has a reserve of bioenergy, which he needs for a normal existence. This life reserve of bioenergy is also called prana.

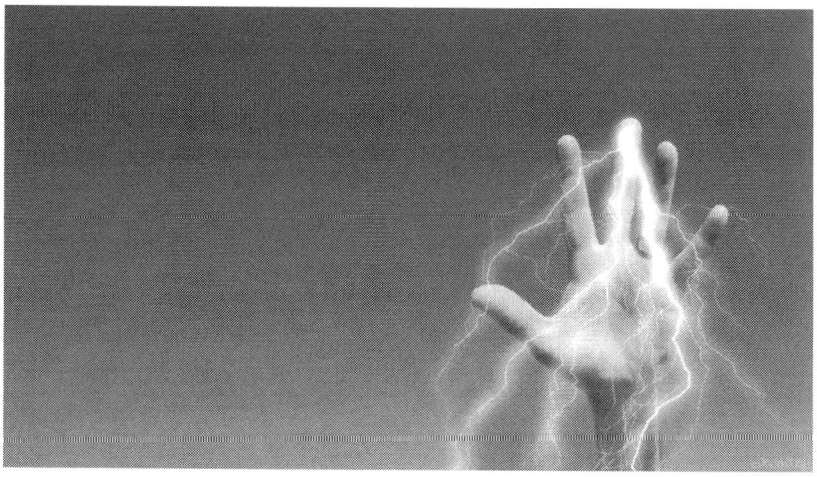

Figure 3. *The cells of the human body radiate energy, this is the human biofield.*

A particular interest related to these processes and especially to the presence of the maximum emission peaks placed in the green area of the spectrum is presented by the works of professor Sorin Comoroşan known as the "Comoroşan effect". The biochemical substrate of the bioluminescence mechanism appears to be provided by the oxidation of lipid free radicals and in particular, unsaturated fatty acids as well as their compounds. The dynamics of the process include, at the same time, the participation of aromatic amino acids, albumin, as well as low molecular weight sugars.

However, the latter components have a lower share of participation. The process itself, according to some hypotheses, consists of the formation of chain self-oxidation reactions in the presence of O2 which begins with the production of a peroxide complex. In the absence of bioluminescence activators in the formation medium, the activated products of the reactions (aldehydes, ketones, oxygen, etc.) participate in the bioluminescence phenomenon: $P^* > P + h\nu$, **{Graphic 1}.**

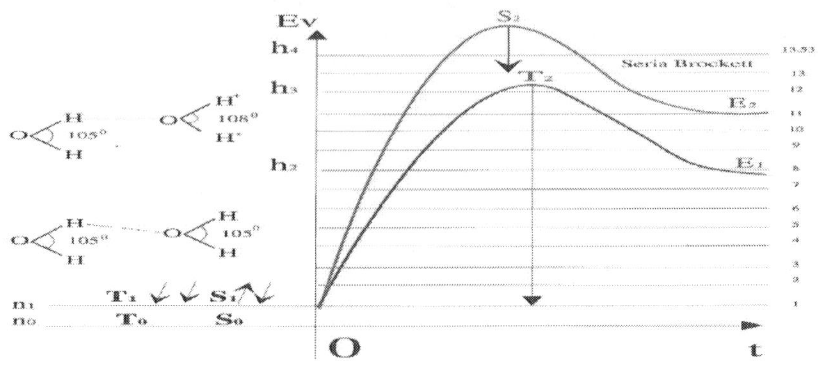

ENERGY OF REVERSE SPIN

Graphic 1. *The bioluminescence phenomenon by emission of photons hv in energetic serry Brockett in atom*

The presence of activators in the molecular state outside the biological structures (ergo-serine, organic amino acids, albumin), is accompanied by their energetic activity and their subsequent transition from the activated state [A *] to the ground state is accompanied by the emission of light quanta:

P * + A ---> P + A * ----P + A + hv

The spectrum of the luminescent emission employing the maximum or part of it on the activator, usually in the area with the longest wavelength.

When subjected to the action of inhibitory radicals or antioxidants, the activators are preserved in the kinetics of the process. The study of the super-weak bioluminescence produced during the process of malignancy by carcinogenic chemicals and in neoplasms with the hormonal substrate (luteomas) showed a decrease in the intensity of cellular bioluminescence. The alteration of the physiological processes of oxidative phosphorylation, the decrease of the respiratory level and the increase of the anaerobic glycolysis in the malignancy processes is accompanied by the decrease of the bioluminescence intensity on the weak cell.

It has been shown by high-sensitivity calorimetric methods that changes in cellular structures at the time of lethal events result in a sudden increase in energy. At the same time, there was a strong burst of light emission over the

weak in the visible range of the spectrum. These data suggest that the changes may be a result of conformational transformations and not only of spontaneous oxidation of lipids as considered, especially when discussing the possible mechanisms for explaining the phenomenon of distant cell death. homologous.

In the para-proximal space, the dissipative process of the energy structure occurs in the form of radiation in different spectral domains. Its usual manifestations can be relatively easily seen in the spectrum of electromagnetic radiation in the IR, visible, UV and RF ranges. The energy dissipation of the biofield can be highlighted by Kirlian procedures, especially in the hypostases of remote interaction in the human-plant and human-human systems. However, the range of field manifestations is much wider, including electromagnetic effects, acoustic effects, magnetohydrodynamic, photoelectric, electromechanical, photonic, chemical, and in the opinion of other authors even types of energy still undiscovered.

The study of Kirlian-type electron-graphy in the clinical diagnosis of cancer has concerned many authors, the first of which belonged to a team of A. Mulatova, R. Stepanov, S.D. Kirlian, V.H. Kirlian. The authors investigated the architecture of the halos formed during the Kirlian procedure, applied to samples of the normal gastric mucosa compared to the pathological one.

The structure described by the electrographic fingerprints, left by the samples of neoplastic gastric mucosa, has as its main element the presence of "penetrations" suggesting micro diffusion processes of IT discharges, in the form of fine globular formations, white or with a grey tint. The same dominant pattern of micro diffusion discharges occurs in lymphoid tissues collected from lymph node areas invaded by metastases. In the case of polyps as opposed to cancerous gastric tissues, there are multiple and massive clusters of discharge channels with a grey tint of fingerprints, which suggests a low conductivity of the tissues.

Electron-graphy is becoming a method of investigation, especially biomedical, thanks to its fundamental property of highlighting the energetic aspects of bio-field phenomena throughout the body, as a result of a resonant response from it to the impulse administered. Among the first uses of electron-graphy as a method of investigation of biological organisms was the exploitation of experimentally induced tumors. The study was performed in comparison with healthy animals and animals with inflammatory processes. The obtained electron-graphic images were compared with the anatomic-pathological picture. At the beginning of the research, the technique of high

voltage and high-intensity electron-graphy was used. In this procedure, the images of the obtained fingerprints show an area of increase of the luminescent emission on the entire projection surface of the neoplastic process. In contrast to this picture, the projection area of inflammatory processes appears as an opaque imprint.

A very special picture is provided by the electrographs made with this technique, to the mice inoculated with murine leukemia. On electrographs, the whole body emits a very strong luminescence, creating the impression of an "incandescence", the electro-morph structure generated by the bloodstream dominating the entire picture of the fingerprint.

Due to the accuracy of the method and the fact that it allows the detection of symptoms that other clinical investigation procedures cannot reveal, electron-graphy can provide serious support in establishing a definite diagnosis of cancer. It reveals your contribution, especially in the follow-up of the post-operative evolution as well as in the follow-up of the appearance and development of metastatic foci, the efficiency of the administered treatments, in the differential diagnosis between inflammation and tumors. Super-weak bioluminescence thus appears as an intrinsic component of metabolism and not as the product of specialized photogenic organs. The loss of cellular bioluminescence, including cellular bioenergy, is equivalent to "raising the soul to the sky" and corresponds to the weight loss of the lifeless body (approximately 21 gr.), [4].

CHAPTER V

BIOENERGETICS OF THE MALIGNANT CELL

Each cell needs the energy to maintain its vital structure, synthesize reserve substances and perform various specific cellular functions and various processes of movement (plasma movement, nuclear and cellular division). As in normal cells, the energy-generating substances are first of all carbohydrates, then fats and proteins, but the use of these principles is done in varying proportions.

Intra-structural and biochemical changes in malignant cells will affect the development of characteristic bioenergetic processes that in turn will condition the expression of cellular oncogenes to the detriment of any oncogenes that are expressed to date, normally in aerobic metabolism. Mitochondrial degeneration frequently occurs in malignant cells. These degenerate mitochondria, which are often found alongside completely normal mitochondria, sometimes have perforated membranes in electron microscopy.

The interior of the altered mitochondria is filled with irregular masses of granular material The progressive increase in the density of the content of these degenerate mitochondria is the expression of an increased amount of intramitochondrial substance. Altered mitochondria are larger. This oversizing should often be attributed to intense, degenerative bloating, when the contents of the mitochondria appear brightly lit and unstructured and very short crystals are highlighted in their lumen.

An accumulation of fatty droplets in the mitochondria has also been observed. Degenerative decomposition, lipid degradation processes and bladder ballooning can be caused by various chemical toxins. Remaining only with these investigations we realize that the possibility of specificity of the mitochondrial changes described during the tumor process is limited.

There is an increase in protein content in the cell nucleus in parallel with an increase in DNA, which occurs during the precancerous state as a radioenzymatic marker. The RNA / DNA ratio is also increased in the nucleus. Malignant tumor proteins have a high characteristic content of D-

amino acids, especially in D-glutamic acid, which by conversion to glutamine participates in the synthesis of nucleic acids. Carcinogens are preferentially stored in lipid-rich cellular structures.

The cytoplasmic structures have a high phosphoprotein content. In the intact tumor cell, with various vital properties of rapid development, a large amount of lecithin is found. Malignant tumors usually contain a higher amount of cholesterol than normal tissues, which according to research by Bierich and others, could evolve in parallel with the degree of malignancy. n many tumors, and especially in poorly irrigated areas, there are accumulations in the form of fat droplets. The cause of these fatty degenerations may be a decrease in the respiratory activity of the cells. Glycogen, as a form of carbohydrate storage in the animal body, is represented in all cells of the body.

A marked increase in glycogen content in tumor tissue was noted. Glucose storage in tumors has never been found, which is explained by an increased degradation of sugar by cleavage, while increasing levels of pyruvic acid --> lactic acid. <--(200-800 μM / 100 gr. Tissue). The increase in the amount of lactic acid due to intense glycolysis causes an increase in the concentration of H + ions in the tumor cell. The pH dependence of various enzymatic functions may be important for metabolic processes.

The cancerous process leads to a general vitamin deficiency of the cells, sometimes very marked. In normal cells, vitamins act mostly in the form of co-ferments (vitamin B1, B2, B6, pantotemic acid, E, K). Vitamins A, C are closely related to the redox processes of the cell and thus take part on a larger scale in respiratory activity. In contrast, folic acid, aspartic, inositol, are generally found in considerable amounts in tumors, sometimes even in cones (> than in normal tissues).

Phosphatases are known to cleave esters of various types of phosphoric acid into alcohol and phosphoric acid. The activity of acid phosphatases is usually low in neoplastic tissues compared to normal T tissues except for prostate cancer where its activity is very high. Alkaline phosphatases in contrast to acid phosphatases are elevated considerably, rarely oscillating with normal values.

Glucose-6-phosphatase is greatly diminished or completely absent in parallel with fructose 1,6-diphosphatase. These findings are of great significance in the diminished gluconeogenesis of tumor tissue. Their activity is the basis of one of the mechanisms of control of carbohydrate

metabolism. B-glycero-phosphatase is 50% lower in tumor tissue than normal. Pyrophosphatase - the activity of this enzyme at pH 6.8 is slightly lower in tumor tissue.

The enzyme adenosine triphosphate (ATPase) hydrolyzes ATP to ADP + Pi. The released energy is usually used for the activity of a substrate to be metabolized. The activity of ATPase in tumor tissue is 40% less than that of normal tissue. This loss of action is mainly attributed to decreased activity of mitochondrial ATPase in the tumor. In the normal liver of the mouse, the activity of ATPase is particularly rich in the nuclear and mitochondrial fraction, while in the hepatoma the highest values of ATPase activity were found in the nuclei and in the fractions of microsomes. Reid and O'Neal found a decrease in "total" ATPase per mg / tissue in liver mitochondria, hepatomas and preneoplasia.

The authors instead observed an increase in free ATPase. Regarding free ATPase, it should be noted that its activity is very low in structurally intact cells. This "active" fraction of ATPase, which in the hepatoma cell appears to be increased relative to the entire ATPase activity, is called latent ATPase. Activation of latent ATPase can be triggered by the various influences exerted on the cell causing structural damage, especially in the mitochondria. Nucleic acid phosphatases and phospho-nucleotides are increased in parallel with the intensity of metabolic processes. In general, the incorporation of amino acids, purine and pyrimidine bases, as well as hexoses and degradation products is considerably increased in the proteins and nucleic acids of malignant tumors.

Glycolysis on the pentose-phosphate pathway as well as on the anaerobic pathway ensures the synthesis of ribozo-5-P, the precursor of PRPP. Xanthin-oxidase - the enzyme that limits the rate of IMP catabolism is 2-10 times lower in all hepatomas. In this way, reprogramming gene expression in neoplastic cells causes an increased capacity for ademin-nucleotide biosynthesis, and excess AMP can be channeled to IMP.

AMP-desaminase which converts AMP to IMP increases in parallel with tumor growth rate but ATPase activity Na, K dependence decreases. Membrane metabolism cAMP -> AMP increases. In this way, cAMP appears low in the cancer cell. Key glycolytic enzymes, hexokinase (HK), phosphofructokinase (PFK) and pyruvate kinase (PK), have been found to increase as liver tumor growth and differentiation increase.

Pyruvate kinase is a key enzyme that acts at an important branching point in glucose metabolism. Strongly allosteric adult hepatic isoenzyme, stimulated by fructose-1,6-diphosphate aldolase and inhibited by ATP, responds to regulation by dietary carbohydrates or hormonal action (insulin).

The lethal hepatic-tumor isoenzyme in contrast to this does not control the host (diet and hormones) or allosteric regulation and has very high enzymatic activity. Pyruvate kinase normally requires ADP from mitochondrial oxidative phosphorylation. Because respiration is closely linked to the phosphorylation of ADP to ATP, pyruvate kinase-dependent glycolysis will be lowered under aerobic conditions, giving rise to the Pasteur effect.

Similarly, the fatal iso-enzymatic type of pyruvate kinase in the tumor may successfully compete for ADP with mitochondrial oxidative phosphorylation, resulting in increased anaerobic glycolysis of the liver tumor. Following the malignant transformation of cells by oncogenic viruses we can distinguish the following biochemical changes: the transformed cells show increased glycolytic activity, protease of hyaluronate synthesis, decreased concentration of AMP (being widely used). cell survival), as well as due to decreased ATP-ase enzyme activity, a change in glycoprotein composition, fetal antigens appear.

In the metabolism of purine-nucleotides, starting from pyrosyl (PRPP) is produced as a key metabolite EVIP - inosinic acid. From EVIP a pathway leads to the de novo synthesis of AMP - ADP - ATP, and a pathway to IMP -> GMP and GTP under the action of the enzymes adenyl succinate-synthetase and GMP synthetase, respectively. In assessing the enzymatic values in the blood, the direct influences of the tumor on the blood must be separated on the one hand, in the sense of the increased presence of certain products released in the blood circulation, and on the other hand the indirect actions in the sense of a system effect.

In addition to disorders of the local tumor metabolism, there is always a disorder of the whole body. This disorder manifests itself in the form of biochemical changes or abnormal immune reactions, as well as in the form of a hormonal imbalance, especially in the various tumors of the endocrine glands.

All these direct or indirect disorders caused by the existence of the tumor, complexes of different nature condition the existence of the patient with the tumor and lead to his death. Example:

• increase in serum LDH in neoplastic patients especially in leukemia and their decrease after tumor regression;

• the appearance of acid phosphatase in metastatic prostate and FAL carcinomas in the serum of patients with osteogenic sarcomas and bone metastases;

• Massive decrease in serum esterase and lipase in cancer patients should be seen as a change in the sense of a systemic effect.

Because these enzymes form in the liver, liver damage can be explained as a consequence of the distant action of tumors. Proteo-lysine and plasmin (prostheses and peptidases) are also elevated in cancer. Free amino acids: tryptophan, tyrosine, phenyl-alanine are increased in the blood plasma although the corresponding enzymes in the liver of leukemic rats are normal. The appearance of lactic acid in the blood should be seen as an expression of intense glycolysis in tumors.

Blood lactic acid has been shown to increase in tumor-bearing animals if given glucose. Chicken myeloblastosis virus obtained by sedimentation methods stimulates the anaerobic glycolysis of a tumor extract isolated with the high speed of centrifugation, which must be attributed to the ATP-ase activity of these particles. One might imagine that due to these presences, structural lesions of the mitochondria appear. The intra-cellular presence of the virus, as a foreign element being at the same time a new genetic layer, influences both the metabolism and the malignant cell division.

The common denominator of malignant degradation due to a virus on the one hand or due to a chemical or physical carcinogen on the other hand, is that in both cases a new genetic substrate appears in the cell in an active form and thus an amplification takes place. Metabolic. Metabolic structural damage of this kind causes metabolic changes of various types, including increased glycolysis by altering intracellular ATP-ase activity.

The hypothesis of the endogenous nature of tumor viruses was one of the theoretical explanations for carcinogenesis. The oncogenic virus under the action of a carcinogen (physical, chemical, biological) causes the modification of the hereditary cellular elements and at the same time of an important metabolic structure.

In parallel, the inhibition of cellular respiration could take place with the activation of glycolysis, which, exceeding the normal physiological intensity and the period of the cell's native resistance, determines the

establishment of malignancy. There are also a number of carcinogens that can directly damage your breath.

Carcinogenic hydrocarbons can accumulate particularly intensely in the mitochondria carrying cellular respiratory enzymes. A particularly strong inhibition is the degradation of glutamic acid, therefore the substance with a key position in the synthesis and degradation of proteins. The higher the malignancy, the lower the tumor respiration and the more intense their glycolysis. In the field of viral oncogenesis in recent years, research has focused on two main directions, namely: the functions of proteins encoded by "v-oc" genes that are responsible for malignant cell transformation and the mechanisms by which cellular oncogene activation (C-onc) is achieved).

To date, three types of transforming proteins have been identified: • tyrosine kinase;

• phosphoprotein kinase;

• proteins that bind to cellular DNA.

Tyrosine kinases are proteins with enzymatic activities that transfer a phosphate from ATP (or GPT) to a protein, thus phosphorylating the protein to tyrosine acid. Tyrosine phosphorylation is a feature because known cellular protein kinases phosphorylate proteins in either serine or threonine or histidine. In recent years, it has been found that cell differentiation is under the control of enzymes that phosphorylate and dephosphorylate proteins, in other words protein kinase and protein phosphatase, respectively.

The ABL oncogene under the action of exogenous-endogenous stimuli destabilizes cell populations through their product phospho-rilate-kinase, an enzyme that phosphorylates triosin residues in various cells (leukemias). A number of normal cell growth factors also act through protein kinases. Oncogenic viral genes synthesize aberrant growth factors that trigger uncontrolled continuous proliferation.

Another control mechanism that can influence the expression of several different genes is represented by the so-called catabolism repression. In essence, the transcription of such genes has been shown to require, in addition to -RNA polymerase, the intervention of specific proteins (cAMP receptor protein) that become active upon interaction with cAMP. CAMP plays an integral role in modulating cell growth and morphology, in the sense that malignant cell division occurs at low levels of cAMP

concentration, while normal differentiation is always associated with high levels of cAMP.

Mg2 + AMP c + H2O ....AMP + H + AMP
phosphodiesterase

Some authors have obtained inhibition of neoplastic tumor by administering cAMP + theophylline. In vitro in the presence of cAMP neoplastic cells returned to normal (Johnson, 1975). Metabolic activation of carcinogenic molecules, initiation, promotion and growth rate are associated with changes in the cyclic intracellular concentration of cAMP in inverse relationship to cGMP. From this information we can say that cancer is a disease of gene disorder and involves the malfunction of complex mechanisms that determine the expression of genes in a given cell in a given time and way of life (Stein et al. 1976).

Disruption of these mechanisms would allow depression or repression of genes in a way not found in normal differential cells. A In determining the functional and structural properties of the genome, it has been shown that nuclear proteins, histones, act as nonspecific repressors of DNA dependent RNA synthesis.

In contrast, non- historic nuclear proteins (NHCPs) contain some components that appear to regulate the transmission of particular genetic sequences. NHCP phosphorylation has been heavily implicated in gene transmission. NHCP phosphorylation is determined by both types of protein kinases: cAMP-dependent and cAMP-independent. Weber (1977) considered that the regulation of gene expression and the reprogramming of their expression in neoplasia are exercised by key enzymes.

In liver cells, enzymatic alterations related to the progression of neoplasia result in an increase in key, glycolytic enzymes, a decrease in key enzymes due to glycogenesis and a change in the iso-enzymatic profile. Deoxy-nucleoside triphosphates including d-ATP have a direct influence on the initiation of DNA synthesis, but also an indirect influence, via allosteric effects, being suggested by the general parallelism between the rate of cell proliferation on the one hand and the cellular reserves of d-ATP and of their synthesis, on the other hand (Canellakis, 1962). An extremely important role in all cellular interactions with the outside, both in direct intercellular contacts and in the mechanism of action of chemical mediators, belongs to the cell membrane.

This membrane is a mosaic of different enzyme systems that selectively allow certain effector molecules to enter or leave the cell, or that lead to the synthesis of secondary messages inside the cell that somehow modulate the processes in the cell. inside the cell. One such secondary message is cAMP.

There is a difference in electrical potential between the cell membrane and the external environment, the decrease in absolute value of which seems to be correlated with an increase in the rate of proliferation (Cone, 1970). The existence of certain receptors on the cell surface and their accessibility are related to the malignant transformations of some cells under the action of DNA viruses or chemicals.

Aggregation of the same malignant cells and regrouping of different normal cell mixtures is also a property of the cell membrane. This mixing of different cells could be explained by a similar calculation of the adhesion and electrostatic repulsion energy between cell pairs. Changes in the cell membrane also mean the loss of contact inhibition by the malignant cell (Burger, 1970).

In addition to changes in electrical potential (±), there is an increase in electrical resistance, which is not seen in rapidly proliferating cells. These membrane transformations also refer to the appearance of specific tumor antigens (Hood, 1972). The body's antibody response, although it appears to be somewhat effective, is too weak due to embryonic tumor antigens, absent in the mature body but re-exposed through malignancy.

The viral oncogenesis model having as its agent transformed the S.V. 40 supports the high incidence of chromosomal aberrations, the hypothesis of somatic mutation as a mechanism of production of neoplastic cells. Cole and Nowel (1965) proposed a multifactorial conception of carcinogenesis that postulates that a tumor is caused by at least two events:

• a mutation;

• a stimulus of cell division.

Cells with micro-structural arrangements in which the mutational process has altered portions of the cell genome with a role in controlling cell division will form the population of transformed cells. Following the events following the penetration of the oncogenic virus into the cell, integration into the cell genome or hybridization of the cellular DNA is the time that appears to initiate a chain of changes in transformation.

For oncogenic viruses - RNA reverses transcriptase in oncogenic DNA transformation. This integration of the oncogenic virus would take place in special sites represented by repetitive nucleotides DNA sequences and would trigger the repression of ancestral oncogenes and also trigger cellular activities preparatory to cell division such as increased syntheses of previously presented cellular enzymes related to DNA replication and cellular DNA synthesis.

The carcinogenetic process results in a higher energy gain of the tumor cell in glycolysis than in respiration if we consider free energy (AE) because the relationship between free energy and that bound in the form of ATP is higher in glycolysis than in glycolysis. oxidation. It is possible that this amount of energy plays an important role for the tumor cell, possibly in the form of increased energy release, which could be related to the increased protoplasmic movement of the tumor cell.

At the same time, the increased amount of ATP resulting from anaerobic glycolysis should be considered as a consequence of the fact that tumor cells can survive longer based on this excess energy, even under anaerobic conditions, in the presence of glucose, unlike normal cells, which die under the same conditions. very fast. This feature gives the tumor cell the ability to survive in the body in unfavorable conditions, especially when there is an insufficient supply of O2. The growth energy of the tumor cell obviously consists of the energy of glycolysis and respiration, while the energy of glycolysis is sufficient to maintain its viability.

Normal cells appear to be dependent on respiration energy for both growth and maintenance. Warburg viewed impaired respiratory function not only as a metabolic symptom of the malignant cell but as a primary cause of malignant degeneration. In his opinion, the action of carcinogenic toxins consisting of an irreversible damage to the activity of cellular respiratory function results in increased glycolysis. Warburg understood by impaired respiration not only a low O2 consumption, but he also took into account the degree of use of O2 to obtain energy.

According to Warburg, this meant that the breath is always damaged when too little ATP is released by oxidative phosphorylation. After damage to the respiration, which causes the migration of ADP and Pi from the mitochondria into the glycolysis space, glycolysis is stimulated, which causes a reversal of the Pasteur effect by tumor pyruvat-kinase.

The importance of glycolysis for the tumor cell can be seen from several points of view:

• glycolysis is the essential energy source for various intense endergonic metabolic processes of the tumor cell;

• by high reserve ATP, during glycolysis, in the presence of glucose, tumor cells incorporate labeled amino acids and sugar into proteins and their nucleic acids, to the same extent as under aerobic conditions, while in the absence of glucose and O2, these synthesis processes are directly stopped;

• constituent elements are provided for different syntheses within the cell growth process. The constituent elements result mainly from the ratio between glycolysis and respiration. Among the metabolic changes in the tumor cells can also list:

a) stimulating the synthesis of amino acids from keto acids;

b) transformation of folic acid into tetra-hydrofolic acid and formyl-tetra-hydro-folic acid and hydroxy-methyl-tetra-hydro-folic acid, up to DNA synthesis, intensifying cell division and growth;

c) increase of RNA synthesis by modifying the ratio of ribose to deoxyribose and NAD synthesis.

d) increasing the glutamine synthesis required for cell division;

e) increase of lactic acid synthesis with extracellular effects to increase tumor vascularization.

In favor of the opinion that in carcinogenesis there would be the primary damage of respiration there are also findings of diminution of various enzymes and coenzymes that participate in respiration: oxidase, cytochrome, dehydrase, flavin-enzymes, DNP, TPN. Some authors believe that in carcinogenesis a primary increase in glycolysis in the cellular regulatory mechanism would be conditioned by the adenyl system. This opinion is also supported by the fact that in some tumors it was not possible to observe a decrease in respiration measured by the consumption of O2 in the tissues.

What is certain is that glycolysis can be inhibited both by the lack of ATP, which is necessary for the initial phosphorylation of glucose, and by the lack of ATP as a phosphate acceptor (di-phosphorylation of di-phospho-glyceric

acid and phospho-enol pyruvic acid) and especially by the lack of inorganic phosphate, formation of triose-diphosphate).

The increase in glycolysis can also be interpreted by the intense increase in the synthesis of ADP and Pi. At the normal cellular level, mitochondria have an equilibrium between ADP, ATP and Pi, which makes optimal glycolysis possible. n normal cells, in which mitochondrial ATPase is completely latent, the glycolysis process is inhibited very effectively. In the tumor cell, according to research by various authors, the intracellular activity of mitochondrial ATPase appears to be increased, which can be deduced from the visible morphological alterations of these organs.

The rapid division of the tumor cell can be explained by the interaction between the electrostatic force (repulsing the global charge of the cell), and the osmatic pressure inside the cell, seeking to increase the cell membrane surface, and the surface tension that seeks to reduce this surface. If the cell grows, it can be shown that when it reaches an uncritical size, the cell will divide.

In the case of some phage DNA, some proteins necessary for replication have been isolated and specifically linked to the AD of these phages (the proteins of gene 12 and gene 32 for phage but also of gene 5 for phage). These proteins bind cooperatively to the phage DNA and mobilize its double helix, making it probably accessible to DNA polymerase.

There is also a need for a threshold amount to start replication and the mechanism for ensuring the exact replication of the entire chromosome. At the base of the carcinogenesis theory exposed so far are the bi-structural and bioenergetic changes of the malignant cell:

- **volume = 4 x 10^{-9} μ^3, compared to normal, (n), 1.5 x 10^{-10} μ^3**
- **protein = 7 x 10^{-10} g /cell, n = 3 x 10^{-11} g /cell**
- **RNA = 6 x 10^{11}, n = 1.3 x 10^{12}**
- **Ribosomes = 1 x 10^{7}, n = 2.5 x 10^{5}**
- **Mitochondria = 1 x 10^{4}, n = 1 x 10^{15}**
- **ATP (molecules / cell / hour) = 2.6 x 10^{12}, n = 3 x 10^{10}. (Kai, 1968).**

If the toxic factors are the very intense, they completely inhibit the respiration and the cell dies in a short time. If these factors are of lower

intensity but act for a long time, cellular respiration may still continue to produce caloric energy instead of lower mitochondrial ATP than glycolytic ATP intensified by toxic influences.

The intimate mechanism of these malignant transformations is not yet well known. Increasing the production of micromolecular precursors may reduce competition between the syntheses of different control proteins over the synthesis of proteins involved in molecular proliferation. The experimental facts seem to be best explained by the hypothesis of an active removal of chalons from the tumor cell which would involve a change in the active transport properties of the cell membrane during malignancy.

In the normal cell, chalons oppose anarchic cell division. Cancer cells differ from normal cells in that they do not synthesize chalona R2 (Operon OF-defect). After increasing the total number of N cells and the position of the cancer cell in the row of N cells (middle or right-left), this cell may be in a state of "rest" (with sufficient R3 concentration, ensured by the other cells by bio-field influences), or may begin to proliferate permanently under the influence of chalone tissue, more or less damaged, depending on the concentration of carcinogens, dispersed intracellularly.

Then the cells no longer synthesize chalone to regulate normal cell division. Elevated aerobic glycolysis in benign hyper-catalytic states may increase the concentration of chalone required to stop uncontrolled proliferation. Oncology experiments to date have shown that the primary effects of carcinogenesis are partial destruction of mitochondrial function followed by early death of a large number of cells and increased rate of renewal and the development of hyperplasia in the direction of malignancy. Another cellular defense factor against carcinogenesis is tumor necrosis factor (TNF).

U.S. researchers at the National Institutes of Health (NIH) have been able to isolate TNF-producing genes and introduce them into a culture of interlenkin-2-stimulated tumor lymphocytes. TNF thus manipulated is transfused to patients. Doctors hope that it will localize in the cancer cells and dissolve the tumor or stop its growth (Steven A. Rosenberg, 1990). The medical world is looking forward to the definite results in the full diversity of neoplasia.

Following extensive research in 1975, Caris Well and colleagues were able to isolate a factor they call "tumor necrosis factor" (TNF) because it causes hemorrhagic necrosis of mouse sarcoma. Its source is also established. It is developed primarily by activated macrophages, then by T and B lymphocytes,

especially the "natural killer" (NK) subgroup. In recent years TNF has been purified: molecular weight 17,000. It is encoded by the gene on the short arm of chromosome 6 in the area of lymphotoxins, more precisely in the histo-compatibility sector (genes of the MHC class l) complex. TNF in the normal body intervenes in inflammatory reactions, activates the metabolism of arachidonic acid and releases prostaglandins. Helps heal wounds by stimulating collagen synthesis.

Participates in immune reactions:

1. activates the phagocytic potential and the production of bactericidal free radicals, the release of antibodies by granulocytes, intensifies the toxic, tumoricidal function. TNF has been shown to be the effector, cytotoxic molecule of "naturally killer" granulocytes and lymphocytes, which are involved in antitumor defense. TNF activates effector T lymphocytes, modulating the production of interferon gamma and interleukin.

2. By enhancing the expression of antigens and molecules of the major histocompatibility system (MHC) in monocytes, endothelial cells, lymphocytes, neutrophil leukocytes, as in tumor cells, it ensures better recognition of foreign elements in the body, harmful, in order to trigger a response. It inhibits the activity of lipoprotein lipase and causes hyperglyceridemia, phenomena previously described as characteristic of casein. TNF obtained by genetic recombination exhibits the same cytostatic and cytotoxic action on tumor cell lines as natural TNF.

Of current interest are its tumoral-toxic properties:

a) on cell proliferation: • in vivo: hemorrhagic necrosis, tumor regression; • in vitro: cytostatic, cytotoxic effect; • inhibiting the development of malignant hematopoietic cells; • tumoral-toxic activation of monocytes; • activation of granulocytes in cytotoxic function, by developing antibodies and producing free radicals (hydroxyl super-oxidation),

b) induction and production of other cytokines such as interleukin 1, interferon gamma, developed by monocytes, T lymphocytes, endothelial cells and fibroblasts. In fact, the invasion of the body by toxins of gram-negative bacteria is responsible for endotoxin shock with cardiovascular collapse. Bacterio-saccharides released by bacteria have been found to induce the production of Tumoral necrosis factor, (TNF).

Other rare side effects of TNF are dizziness, vomiting, soft stools, and muscle aches. The antitumor effect marked by tumor regression! ranges

from 10-20%. The best effects have been reported in colorectal cancer and kidney tumors. We have at our disposal two immuno-stimulating preparations of bacterial origin, with antitumor activity mediated by TNF and interferon gamma. Drug product by the Cantacuzino Institute, Cantastim vaccine, (Dr. A. Olinescu), justify to use by the results obtained on the residual disease (tumor residue after surgical removal, radio and chemotherapy).

Survival is definitely prolonged, metastasis is avoided. The effects on solid tumors are very limited. Attempts to increase the dose of TNF to intensify its effects are hindered by the violence of side effects. It seems that the combination of cortisone would reduce the intensity of the reactions. Broncho-vaxone is expected to increase antitumor effects. It stimulates the body's defense system and increases resistance to respiratory tract infections (Labor Geneva).

This effect has been demonstrated by stimulating macrophages and increasing the number of circulating T lymphocytes as well as immunoglobulins produced in the mucous membranes of the respiratory tract. In cases of severe human immunodeficiency with T4 lymphocytes below 2000 (AIDS), the first drug that prolongs the irreversible evolution of AIDS by 10 months, Zidovudine (Azidothymidine), has been discovered. Being an artificially created nucleotide, it replaces those of the HIV virus itself, blocking its multiplication.

The genetic substance is made up of small molecular fragments - nucleotides, composed of a nitrogenous base (ex, cytosine, tymine, uracil), a sugar (a pentose). Folk medicine claims that there are teas that can cure cancer. In fact, these toxic and medicinal plant infusions, through the lectins they contain, could activate cellular TNF.

After their gradual administration, in order for the body to adapt to the drug, the patients presented symptoms similar to the administration of high doses of TNF: myalgias, low back pain, nausea, dizziness, lack of strength, bioenergy. Following their progressive administration up to 100 ml There have been cases of patients cured, even with metastases, within 2-3 months of starting administration.

Lectin oligosaccharide receptors are randomly and diffusely distributed on the surface of normal or malignantly transformed cells. The addition of a lectin with several combination sites interconnects the receptors, aggregating them progressively, forming "caps". The formation of "caps" requires

energy consumption and involves the transmission of signals from the cell membrane to the nucleus through the activity of contractile microfilaments. Through these signals also takes place the redistribution of a protein located on the inner surface of the cell membrane, spectrin.

Spectrin, being in contact with the cytoplasm and through it with the cell nuclei, could influence the course of the cellular "machinery" and its activity. In parallel, the activation of adenylate cyclase and the increase of cellular cAMP with the role of inhibitor of cellular mitosis, modification of carbohydrate metabolism, transmethylation of membrane lipids, changes in the flow of monovalent ions (K +, Na% Ca2 +), acceleration of protein synthesis, RNA, of polyamines and lymphocytic TNF. Lectins bind to several cell types, but generally have a major characteristic activity.

There are lectins capable of selective binding to both T cells and B lymphocytes. Current antiviral medications are analogs of nucleosides. In order to multiply, retroviruses, the group to which HIV belongs, have a specific enzyme, reverse transcriptase; it converts the nucleic acid in the cytoplasm, ribonucleic acid, into nuclear-type nucleic acid, (deoxyribonucleic acid, DNA), the only one that can degrade viral proliferation. In the presence of zidovudine, the virus uses the false nucleotide instead of its own nucleotide and the multiplication chain is interrupted. Multiple or mixed infection of a single cell, in vivo or in vitro, which leads to the annihilation of the multiplication of a virus, is known as interference and has long been reported by many authors (Isaacs and Sindenman, 1957).

These authors have shown that the particle interference does not directly cause changes in the host cell but through an environmentally diffuse factor called interferon. In this sense, interferons have been considered today as cytokines, ie proteins that carry important chemical messages in regulating the functions of various cells in the body. Because cytokines are cell-released mediators that influence the function of other cells and interferons, they are a system of communication between all nucleated cells in the body.

Interferon is a cellular protein that is only synthesized in the presence of a stimulus represented by a virus or other non-viral inducers. During the stages of the virus's multiplication, some molecular events (probably the presence of foreign viral acid) disregard a cellular gene that contains genetic information for the interferon protein. Genes for human interferons are found in human chromosomes 2,5 and 9.

Interferon uses secondary messenger molecules to transfer information, both inside the cell and between cells. This system amplifies the interferon system and appears to be the mechanism of spread of anti-viral activity, especially of the avascular tissues (surface of the respiratory tract, gastrointestinal tract and occlusion), and in tissues accessible to mobile leukocytes (local inflammation).

There are a variety of interferon inducers that can be classified into two groups:

1) The first group includes viruses, viral extracts and synthetic polynucleotides that stimulate the production of interferon in all cellular systems, in vivo and in vitro and whose inducing capacity is related to the presence of double RNA.

2) The second group includes heterogeneous inducers such as bacteria, bacteria endotoxins, mitogens (specific and nonspecific), polyanions and single molecular weight compounds. All inducers in the second group are active in vitro or in leukocyte cultures and generally produce lower amounts of interferon. Based on antigenic specificities, a classification of human interferon (Hm-IFN) was made into three distinct types: alpha, beta and gamma.

The first researcher to demonstrate that human leukocytes can be used as a cell substrate for interferon induction was Gresser (1961). Interferon alpha was found in larger quantities using the lymphoblastic cell line (Buckler, 1978). Beta interferon was obtained on human fibroblasts, human diploid line FS-4 or clonal cell line called C-10, derived from human embryonic fibroblasts transformed by SV-40, the interferon obtained on this line is also known as fibroblast interferon.

Due to the potential importance of this type of interferon in the treatment of viruses and neoplastic diseases, different production and purification methods have been studied. Gamma interferon inducers can be classified into several categories, being represented by a variety of antigens, antigens, lymphocyte antibodies, enzymes and mixed lymphocyte reactions. The most commonly used inducers are phyto-hemaglutinina, concavalin A1, staphylococcal enterotoxin, author (Staton, 1985). Interferons have a variety of biological effects, which is why they are considered to have multiple potential regulatory factors. In addition to their role in defending the body against viruses, they have important implications for immunology, cancer, cell genetics, regulation of protein synthesis, and cell differentiation.

The life of organisms depends on the normal functioning of intricate mechanisms, on the intracellular communication through which the metabolic activity of the huge number of cells is coordinated. Induction and active processes of interferon during viral infection are examples of such an intercellular communication system. Because cells communicate with the environment at the cytoplasmic membrane, an important step in understanding the molecular mechanisms of regulatory agents is to elucidate the process of interaction with the cell surface.

The modulating effects of interferon on the cell membrane represent a major step in its regulatory action on the various phenotypic expressions of the cell. This property of interferon is probably one of the main physiological roles. Interferon inhibits early protein synthesis without altering the absorption, penetration, and decapitation of infected virions. Molecular mechanisms underlying interferon-induced antiviral status include: primary inhibition of viral mRNA transcription, post-transcriptional changes in viral mRNA, and inhibition of viral mRNA translation.

Research on the elucidation of the first mechanism has shown that dsRNA (viral or synthetic) inhibits acellular protein synthesis and that the addition of dsRNA, which is an interferon inducer, to interferon-treated cell extracts increases translational inhibition of mRNA. viral. These observations led to the discovery of two interferon-induced enzymes and their dependence on dsRNA and ATP: 2-5 synthetase and protein kinase.

Enzyme 2-5 A synthetase activates cellular endonucleases that leads to viral mRNA degradation and protein kinase phosphorylates in the presence of ATP, which acts as a catalyst for the reaction, the e-F-2 subunit, thus blocking the initiation of protein synthesis. Because the synthesis of these two enzymes is dependent on the presence of ds-RNAs, these molecular species of ds-RNAs are considered to be modulators, ie inducers and activators of the interferon system. They appear as an intermediate in the replication of many viruses and are probably the signal by which the cell monitors the presence of the replicating virus (Sen, 1982).

Admitting that exogenous neoplastic disease is grafted onto an initially healthy organism, we deduce that establishing the body's defense mechanisms in which it is induced and decreasing mitochondrial ATP and increasing cytoplasmic ATP engaged in specific mechanisms of malignant bioenergy in the absence of interferon malignant. Interferons are considered to be the first group of well-characterized molecules that reversibly inhibit cell proliferation. Numerous studies have shown that interferons inhibit the

growth of normal, tumor or transformed cells in vivo and in vitro (Danielescu et al., 1983).

Interferons influence immune responses in vitro and in vivo. Modulation of the immune response by interferon is characterized by suppression or increased humoral immune response, suppression of antigen- or mitogen-induced lymphocyte proliferation, increased ADCC, increased NK cytotoxicity, macrophage activation, and increased specific cytotoxicity of T lymphocytes. The results obtained with human T cells show that gamma (immune) interferon synthesized by specifically sensitized lymphocytes, after a new contact with the same viral antigen, is one of the mediators of cellular immunity to viruses. Immune interferon is therefore a lymphokine produced by TH lymphocytes as a result of immune recognition phenomena. To date, it is the only lymphokine that can exert positive and negative control over the immune system.

Molecular mechanisms underlying interferon-induced antiviral status include: primary inhibition of viral mRNA transcription, post-transcriptional changes in viral mRNA, and inhibition of viral mRNA translation. Research on the elucidation of the first mechanism has shown that dsRNA (viral or synthetic) inhibits acellular protein synthesis and that the addition of dsRNA, which is an interferon inducer, to interferon-treated cell extracts increases translational inhibition of mRNA. viral. T

These observations led to the discovery of two interferon-induced enzymes and their dependence on dsRNA and ATP: 2-5 synthetase and protein kinase. Enzyme 2-5 A synthetase activates cellular endenucleosis leading to viral mRNA degradation and protein kinase phosphorylates in the presence of ATP, which acts as a catalyst for the reaction, the subunit is F-2, thus blocking the initiation of protein synthesis.

Because the synthesis of these two enzymes is dependent on the presence of ds-RNAs, these molecular species of dsRNAs are considered to be modulators, ex. inducers and activators of the interferon system. They appear as an intermediate in the replication of many viruses and are probably the signal by which the cell monitors the presence of the replicating virus (Sen, 1982). Admitting that exogenous neoplastic disease is grafted onto an initially healthy organism, we deduce that establishing the body's defense mechanisms in which it is induced and decreasing mitochondrial ATP and increasing cytoplasmic ATP engaged in specific mechanisms of malignant bioenergy in the absence of interferon malignant.

Interferons are considered to be the first group of well-characterized molecules that reversibly inhibit cell proliferation.

Numerous studies have shown that interferons inhibit the growth of normal, tumor or transformed cells in vivo and in vitro (Danielescu et al., 1983). Interferons influence immune responses in vitro and in vivo. Modulation of the immune response by interferon is characterized by suppression or increased humoral immune response, suppression of antigen- or mitogen-induced lymphocyte proliferation, increased ADCC, increased NK cytotoxicity, macrophage activation, and increased specific cytotoxicity of T lymphocytes.

The results obtained with human T cells show that gamma (immune) interferon synthesized by specifically sensitized lymphocytes, after a new contact with the same viral antigen, is one of the mediators of cellular immunity to viruses. Immune interferon is therefore a lymphokine produced by TH lymphocytes as a result of immune recognition phenomena. To date, it is the only lymphokine that can exert positive and negative control over the immune system. This double effect of interferon is explained on the one hand by the inhibitory effect on lymphocyte proliferation

It is an important phenomenon that underlies the negative control by activating macrophages (Huangri et al., 1975) and phagocytosis, thus increasing the rate of antigen processing by these cells, thus stimulating immune reactions. Natural and recombinant beta interferon, as well as most alpha species (except type J), rapidly and rapidly increase human NK cell activity in vitro (Herberman et al., 1985). Interferon gamma has less known effects on NK activity and requires a longer time for spontaneous cytotoxicity (Smeiero et al., 1981). Experimental data suggest that interferon may act in vitro not only directly by increasing mature cells, but also by inducing the proliferation of these cells indirectly via interleukin 2 (Birou et al., 1983).

Interferon stimulates the activity of NK cells through at least three mechanisms:

1) differentiation of NK precursors;

2) proliferation of mature NK cells;

3) increased cytotoxic activity (Timonem et al., 1952).

The appearance of an interferon-inducing stimulus in a tissue, viral infection or tumor growth (produces higher levels of interferons that induce a sequence of events). NK cells become very active and are able to lyse any type of cell. The interferon protects cells from normal lysis tissue, but because the protective effect is selective, virus-infected or tumor cells are not protected. So the activity of NK cells will be focused on the pathological cells. Consequently, interferon enables the NK system to acquire two characteristics necessary for any effective defense mechanism: induction and selectivity (Trinchieni, 1984). Because there are experimental data on the induction of interferon gamma by IL-2 (Pearlstein, 1983), the relationship between interferon and IL-2 is quite complex considering that interferon induces IL-2 receptors on the surface of NK and IL-2 cells. 2, induces the growth and maturation of NK cells.

Interferons also amplify the expression of MHC class I and II antigens, thus indirectly influencing the antiviral immune response (Rodnes et al., 1983). All types of interferon have an antitumor activity that can be tested in vivo and in vitro in tumor systems, an activity that has been confirmed in preliminary data obtained by administering interferon in human neoplasms.

Interferons have an antitumor effect in vitro or on virus-induced neoplasms, carcinogenic substrate-induced tumors, neoplasms and transplantable tumors. Interferon significantly reduces the incidence of neoplastic (Gresser et al., 1976) and delays the onset of breast tumors provided it is administered intensively and repeatedly (Cone and Moore, 1972).

The action of interferon on the phenotype of malignantly transformed cells, depending on the cell type, is manifested either by complete reversion to the normal phenotype (Gresser et al., 1977) or by partial reversal (Danielescu, 1985). Interferon can also influence the expression of surface cell antigens in tumor cells, thereby influencing their elimination by specific or nonspecific host effector cells. Administration of interferon in breast carcinoma at doses of 3 x IO6 U i.m. for 2 months it resulted in the remission of the tumor in a proportion of 70% of the number of people (Gutterman, 1980).

Recent research has shown that high doses (9 x IO6 U) are more effective than lower doses (3 x IO6 U) in inducing enzymes (2-5 A synthetase) and HLA-DR protein expression in peripheral monocytes as well. stimulation of precursor NK activity (Ment et al., 1985). The analysis of the action of interferons in vivo, situations in which they represent only one component,

from a complete system of intracellular communications, dynamic and complete, is a difficult problem that remains to be clarified by new research.

We have reviewed the above pharmacological means not to propose a new isolated therapy in the field of cancer but to complete the therapeutic regimen of cytostatic after surgical resection of the tumor and radiotherapy; more precisely, after the surgeons finish their work and the patient stays with himself longer. After the initial marked effect of tumor retraction, cytostatic gradually lose their effectiveness.

The malignant tissue becomes more resistant and follows the stage of metastases against which chemotherapy remains ineffective. In 1981, the author Tsurno found an enhanced activity of Vincaprine's Verapamil on leukemia cells. Verapamil opened the series of calcium β-blockers a long time ago. Without possessing its own cytostatic action, Verapamil (Isoptin) intervenes indirectly; amplifies the into-tumoral circulation and thus the concentration of the active substance becomes higher and is retained longer in tumors.

A competitive inhibition of cytostatic elimination of the cell membrane was also found. Another antitumor mechanism has recently been seen. Blockade of the calcium-Colmodulin complex greatly influences many intracellular enzymatic reactions necessary for malignant proliferation. Verapamil is currently expected to be associated with Melphalan in melanoma and Doxirubicin in breast and pancreatic tumors. Reading the neo-therapy of malignancies we may wonder: What is the mechanism by which it would contribute to the inhibition of malignant tumors? We know that the cancer cell needs for its rapid growth and multiplication a large amount of mono-, bi- and triphosphate nucleotides, as well as hormonal stimuli triggered by negative, stressful neuropsychic reactions, hormones that act through membrane structures on secondary messengers. intracellular (cAMP, cCMP, phosphatidyl-inositol-choline).

This link between hormonal stimulation and the synthesis of the second messenger is made by a system that associates cellular receptors, regulatory proteins (R protein, inhibitors or stimulators) and enzymes responsible for the synthesis of the second messenger. Increased intracellular cAMP causes activation of a protein kinase.

This kinase causes the phosphorylation of several membrane proteins, which appear to control the movement of electrolytes in the initially healthy cell. Stimulation of the dependent system is due to the degradation of

phosphatidyl-inositol-choline in a number of secondary metabolites, diacyl-glycerol and inositol-triphosphate.

The first stimulates a protein kinase (protein kinase C) and the second causes a mobilization of intracellular calcium. An important role is played by the calcium transporter protein, calmodulin. Stimulation of these kinases results in a phosphorylation of several membrane proteins that control the movement of electrolytes. The calcium-dependent system acts like various hormonal or neurotransmitter substances, acetylcholine, norepinephrine, somatostatin, or substance P.

Acetylcholine stimulates non-electrogenic absorption of Ca. Noradrenaline increases cAMP and calcium. That's why positive emotions, joy, and happiness increase our resilience. Somatostatin decreases intracellular cAMP values. Again, the hypothalamic balance makes its mark on health. Substance P, the intestinal cellular polypeptide, increases its secretion, probably by acting on the calcium-dependent system. We cannot conclude with a clear conscience if we do not remember the principles that, according to the specialists gathered under the leadership of Prof. Maurice Tubara, can determine the regression of the current incidence of cancer in Europe:

1). Don't smoke, be careful not to force others to inhale your smoke (bronchopulmonary cancer);

2). Drink less alcohol (risk of esophageal cancer);

3). Do not expose yourself too much to the sun (excess ultraviolet decreases immunity);

4). Follow the advice on work protection and professional activity;

5). Eat more fruits, vegetables, vegetables, plant products rich in fiber (normal digestive transit avoids stagnation of carcinogenic toxins);

6). On the contrary, it reduces the consumption of fat and excess calories, which increases weight (adiposity predisposes to breast cancer through increased estrogen synthesis);

7). Consult your doctor at any change in the configuration of a tumor that is considered benign to abnormal bleeding;

8). Beware when coughing, hoarseness, unexplained weight loss, intestinal dysfunction (constipation, less often diarrhea) persistent;

9). Regular monitoring of the breasts in women and the general condition of men, considering that women have a native predisposition for the figure and for the factors that increase their health and beauty, [5].

Chapter VI

Significance of the ATP-Mg complex in experimental papers

Mitochondrial contraction and ballooning have been the subject of various investigations in specialized laboratories. Despite detailed knowledge of the conditions that induce or inhibit ballooning, the mechanism of this process has not yet been clearly explained. The changes in the volume of the mitochondria are based on two phenomena:

1. the change in the volume of the mitochondria can be given by the transport of ions that cause the osmotic and water transport;

2. The change in volume of the mitochondria can also be initiated by the mechano-chemical or conformational transformation of the mitochondrial membrane with ATP consumption, thus creating differences in hydrostatic pressures that develop in the system. Research has shown that oxidized substances through the respiratory chain increase ballooned mitochondria, while components that inhibit electron transport counteract this effect.

It has been established that ballooning is thus dependent on electron transport. Ballooning occurs more rapidly in the presence of oxygen than in anaerobiosis with the presence of electron transporter inhibitors. Mitochondrial contraction has been linked to an increase in ADP levels by converting ATP to ADP and thus ballooning can be initiated by the addition of substrate (glutathione, pyruvate) along with ATP in the vicinity of an active ATP-ase. The addition of ATP alone can cause maximal contraction if it is cleaved by ATP-ase into ADP. The presence of added strontium in the ionic reaction medium has the effect of supporting ATP-induced contraction which rapidly converts to ADP. Str2 + can be replaced by Mg2 + without changes in the frequency or extent of contraction.

Experimental data have shown that Ca ions accumulate significantly during ATP contraction, probably due to ATP hydrolysis. Mitochondrial ballooning as a result of aging or the addition of Ca or thyroxine is accompanied by the release of "U" factor or free fatty acids. These in turn can cause the

respiratory chain not to be coupled with oxidative phosphorylation, as the free fatty acids resemble in this action 2,4-dinitrophenol, an inhibitor of oxidative phosphorylation. We also note from research that strontium inhibits the activity of ATP-ase, stimulated by Mg even in aged mitochondria. In fact, this aspect of Mg ATP=ase, activation is a typical criterion for altered mitochondrial structure. The bivalent strontium ion could form bridges between pairs of negatively charged groups in the cell membrane and thus determine the stability of its structure. Positive ions, spermine and spermidine in fruits, can protect the mitochondria against spontaneous, inefficient bloating, can replace Mg as a support for oxidative phosphorylation in microsomal systems (Ishikawa and Lehminger, 1990), **[Scheme 4].**

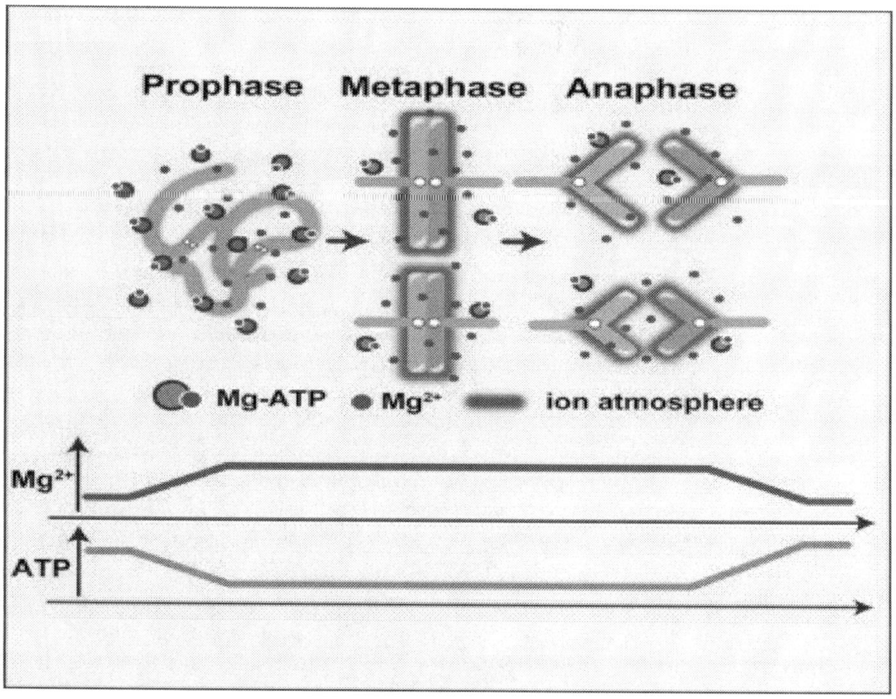

Scheme 4. *Mg ion is a support for oxidative phosphorylation in microsomal systems*

It is assumed that these cations are effective due to the specific spacing of the positive charges on the cell membrane. The stabilizing effects of strontium and Mg and the reverse ballooning action of Ca appear to be a reflection of the size of these ions and their action of spatially dispersing

negative charges on the mitochondrial membrane. Because the reactants (substrate, O2, P and ADP) and oxidative phosphorylation have a characteristic effect on the steady state of mitochondrial contraction, it has been postulated that these metabolites act by affecting a common intermediate.

It has been hypothesized that the regulation of mitochondrial contraction is considered to be governed by the concentration of energy-rich intermediates resulting from oxidative phosphorylation. The influence of pH on mitochondrial ballooning has also been observed under certain experimental conditions. In presence of phosphate the extent of ballooning increases with increasing pH from 5.6-7.5. A higher pH increase causes an increase in the time of onset of bloating. These effects of pH change must be manifested as a such changes in the frequency of enzymatic reactions or as a change in the concentration of ionic species associated with mitochondrial integrity.

Below pH 7.5, where the extent of the ballooning is smaller than the maximum, both respiration and ATP can cause an increase in ballooning. Ballooning appears to be caused by one or more intermediates generated by substrate oxidation in the presence of phosphate and ATP. Antimycin A, which inhibits O10 exchanges in mitochondria in liver cells at pH 8.2, has had only mild inhibitory activity when ATP is present in mitochondria.

At pH 7.4 the protective effect of ATP does not prevent its hydrolysis to Pi or PPi but is proportional to the amount of ATP added. Analysis of the similar effects of ATP and substrate on the ballooning time suggests that these agents act in the same direction, probably causing a change in the balance of reactions that in some way controls the limitation of the ballooning process in experiments performed at pH 7.4.

Huxley's discovery is particularly important: the cleavage of ATP is necessary for the contraction of mitochondria, and the existence of ATP, in conditions where its cleavage cannot occur, causes mitochondrial ballooning. Early investigations showed that ATP, the end product of phosphorylation, acts to delay the mitochondrial ballooning process and even to contract ballooned mitochondria by thyroxine or other agents.

It all depends on the proper functioning of the ATP-aze in the intact mitochondria. Restoration of the mitochondrial ATP pole may even decrease intracellular damage induced by changes in the physicochemical conditions of the internal environment. The results of the research aim at a new trend in the chemotherapy of chronic diseases deficient in ATP, namely

that of associating pharmaceutical drugs with derivatives of ATP (phosphobion) and Mg (ascorbate of Mg).

Following the above experiments, we can imagine the mitochondria as a clock that by a "tac-tic" mechanism marks its contraction - rhythmic ballooning, as long as it - will lose its rhythm of aging or disease.

2. Nutrition, inducing or suppressing factor of carcinogenesis

During its evolution, the human species has created a complex metabolism served by a very diverse enzymatic equipment. Nutrition makes its mark starting with the formation and evolution of the embryo.

The definition of the human phenotype is a complex process in which the essential role is played by hereditary characters that can be influenced by the concrete conditions of the diet. Mathematical models have even been developed to calculate the evolution of the embryo according to genotype, maternal phenotype and feeding characteristics. The decrease in fetal weight is not only caused by involution, as a result of the overall reduction of food but also by dietary imbalances caused by deficiency of proteins, essential fatty acids, amino acids, vitamins and bio-elements. Malnutrition mainly affects the development of the brain, liver, reticulo-endothelial system tissue, blood and heart.

In last years, research conducted in 1939 by McCay has been brought back to life, stating that limiting food intake has favorable effects on longevity. Several studies have found that reducing energy intake has allowed for the prolongation and even doubling of the lives of experimental animals. The phenomenon is associated with slowing down the aging process at different levels of biological organization.

Low-energy animals lower their lipid and cholesterol levels. At the same time, the need for O2 increases, the transformation of DNA into tissues is slowed down, the aging of collagen is stopped, and the acid-base balance is stabilized in the alkaline domain. Prolonged life and conditions of a reduced energy ratio is correlated with inhibiting the aging of the human genome. At the same time, age-induced neuroendocrine changes are inhibited. In the elderly, the need for protein, lipids and carbohydrates decreases, but the need for biocatalysts and antioxidants increases! (ascorbic acid, tocopherols, selenium, methionine, cysteine, polyphenols), which inhibit the reactions of free radicals, responsible for many pathological conditions.

Modern man is deficient in vitamins and minerals. Preferences for white bread, pasta has led to a decrease in the content of Ca, phosphorus, Mg, potassium with a significant increase in sodium assimilation. Research by various authors has shown that energy metabolism is closer in this case to the anaerobic phase, which develops by increasing the content of pyruvic acid in the blood. This phenomenon is accompanied by an increase in the need for vitamins B1 and B6 to restore aerobic metabolism.

Epidemiological studies have shown that people who work under conditions of mental stress need an additional intake of iron and calcium. Therefore, maintaining the homeostasis of the internal environment of the body depends on the nature of the diet that influences the functions of the system, enzymatic and hormonal factors. Insufficiency of a nutrient especially influences the cellular metabolic background.

Thus, energy deficiency causes a decrease in the synthesis of these CoA and ATP syntheses; protein deficiency affects the concentration of free amino acids; avitaminosis leads to a decrease in reserves and a decrease in the concentration of the corresponding coenzymes; the insufficiency of trace elements influences the mineral background of the cell and the organic compounds in the composition of which many of them play an active role.

The deficiency of substances in the food ration, over a determined period of time, in the preclinical stage can be compensated on the basis of biochemical adaptation processes. As a result, the disease sets in when the body's ability to adapt is exhausted and there is an imbalance at the cellular level. A large number of epidemiological studies conducted recently by national and international organizations in many countries are increasingly highlighting the correlation between diet and cancer.

Most current studies show that excessive consumption of food, ingestion of a large the amount of calories is correlated with the occurrence of cancer in both animals and humans. In the particular, increasing the consumption of meat and fat promotes the induction of colon cancer. The US ANS Recommendations on Cancer Prevention can be summarized as follows:

• avoiding overweight and excess calories;

• reduction of fat consumption to 30% of the previous ration, for overweight people;

• reduction of consumption of animal fats (saturated) and compensation by polyunsaturated fats (vegetable origin);

• increase the consumption of carbohydrates from vegetables and fruits, with the reduction of refined carbohydrates;

• increasing the intake of biologically active substances, vitamins and bio-elements. As a result, it is necessary to enrich food with nutrients whose lack has been recorded in the diet of contemporary man.

The influence of diet on thc induction of cancer can be determined by 2 factors:

1. Excessive intake of nutrients, especially proteins and lipids, which are involved in the development of primary cancer;

2. Choline deficiency can lead to liver cancer, and iodine deficiency can induce thyroid cancer. The role of tryptophan, which promotes female sex hormone-induced carcinogenesis, is being monitored. The presence in the food of substances with a direct carcinogenic effect which may exist naturally or as a result of food contamination processes may be associated with the deficiency of the factors listed above and may initiate carcinogenesis.

However, very small doses of carcinogens that cause cancer can only sensitize the body to carcinogens, and depending on the duration of action can have cumulative effects. Polycyclic aromatic hydrocarbons (HPA) are initially chemically inert and therefore require prior metabolic activation to take effect. Epoxides are initially formed, extremely active transient compounds that may be suspected of being responsible for carcinogenic action. These electrophilic compounds can react as cellular constituents such as proteins or nucleic acids. According to the "intercalation" theory, epoxy-filled molecules that occur between two neighboring bases of the DNA molecule can cause a transcription error of a part of the gene. Carcinogenic HPAs are approx. 3.6 A similar to purine and pyrimidine base pairs and may be embedded in the structure of nucleic acids.

Stereochemical similarity also occurs. The electrophilic character of the epoxides ensures the stability of the intercalation with the nucleophilic center of the base, while the flat hydrocarbon molecule does not exert this effect and does not show mutagenic action. In the presence of carcinogenic food compounds, including under the action of HPA, there is a significant increase in the amount of cytochromes P 450 and b 5 in the cell with the intensification of oxidase activity with mixed functions.

Compared to the initiation of carcinogenesis, which is a reversible process due to structural damage to DNA, the promotion of carcinogenesis has been

shown to be a reversible step. The essential role of promotion is to select the "initial" cells, the growth of which stimulates it. Only during the depression of the promotion stage, the cell enters the phase of progression that leads to the formation of the tumor through an irreversible cell development. Increased susceptibility to carcinogens in cells with a low repair capacity for some types of DNA-induced lesions in DNA has been shown.

The interaction of mutagenic chemicals with DNA can lead to alteration of the information contained in the genome by initially modifying the structure of DNA and then the natural sequence of its constituent bases. The least possible alteration, defined as a point mutation, consists structurally in the modification or replacement of a nucleotide (or pair of nucleotides) and is functionally translated by the modification of a codon.

The possibility of fixing and transcribing this change, an essential feature of mutagenesis, is based on the reproductive "safe" character of the DNA molecule. Mutations in a gene can directly or indirectly inactivate the expression of other genes, suspending or inducing mutations (of an enzyme, amino acid, or other enzyme that causes a new metabolic pathway or intensifies existing ones).

In this way, more intense expression of the pentose-phosphate pathway in the cancer cell as well as anaerobic and aerobic ATP synthesis may also occur. For neoplastic transformation, mutation at the level of a regulatory gene appears more important as a biochemical significance than at the level of structural genes. The mutation produced by a chemical can be reversed by other chemicals or even by the same substance through a mutational process.

Regulatory processes can occur that can even repair important DNA damage. Mammalian normal cells have a very active repairing enzyme system, but errors can also be caused by accidents caused by certain unknown microenvironmental conditions. Even the activity of allelic genes for proper RNA synthesis can compensate for the effect of a mutation in a eukaryotic genome. Initially, the body defends itself by biochemical means. Foreign substances - xenobiotics - once produced in the body undergo a complete biotransformation.

The hydroxylation system consists of 3 components:

1. Cytochrome P 450 which is found mostly in the endoplasmic reticulum; 2.

2. NADPH-cytochrome P 450 reductase flavoprotein, which ensures the transport of electrons from NADPH to cytochrome P450; The enzyme is formed from FAD and FMN. 3.
3. Phospholipids (phosphatidylcholine) that participate in the stabilization of the active conformation of cytochrome P 450 and in the process of electron transfer.
4. Deficiency in various dietary factors may be a primary cause of carcinogenesis, **[Scheme 5].**

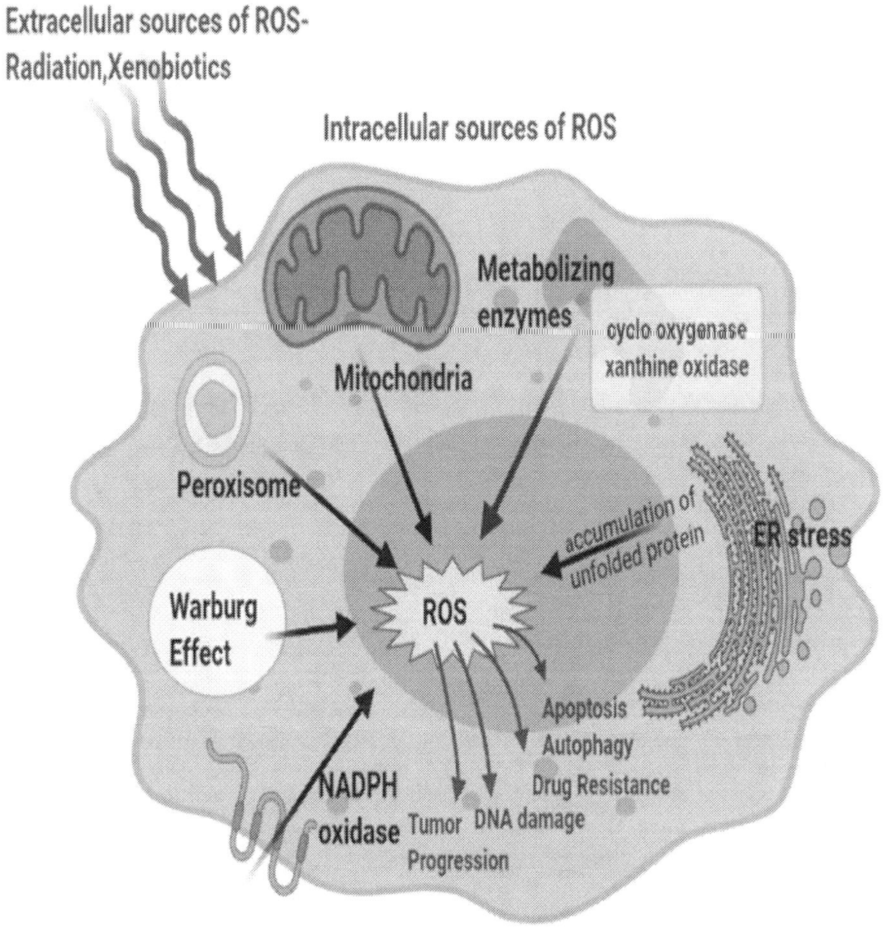

Scheme 5. *Free radicals of oxygen, (ROS) of metabolism from various dietary factors may be a primary cause of carcinogenesis.*

As a result of all these reactions, the fat-soluble compounds become more polar than the initial ones, which ensures their elimination from the body. This is the main function of the microsomal mono-oxidase system. In the process of transforming xenobiotics through the participation of OFEMN, electrophilic metabolites are formed with a high reaction capacity having a carcinogenic and mutagenic activity.

The diet, especially the vegetarian diet, contains compounds that activate the detoxification process, thus performing antimutagenic and anticancer effects. In the vegetarian field, in addition to cabbage, wheat germ, parsley, apples reduce the mutagenic activity of tryptophan. They contain a complex of antioxidants that alter the enzyme system in cell microsomes, which neutralizes mutagenic and carcinogenic substances. Microsomal biotransformation goes through 2 phases: in the first phase under the action of OFMN, xenobiotics gain groups with high reactive capacity so that later in the second phase conjugation reactions with endogenous substrate take place as a result of the formation of reactive groups in the first phase of biotransformation.

They may react by conjugation with endogenous metabolites of glucuronic acid, sulfate, methyl or glycine. An important class of conjugates is sulfuric acid esters that form as a result of the interaction of sulfate with xenobiotics or their metabolites. The synthesis of sulfo-esters is done in several stages:

• at the beginning, adenosine 3-5 phospho-sulfate is synthesized, which in the subsequent stages passes into conjugated compounds;

• Aliphatic foreign substances and aromatic compounds containing 1 electrophilic carbon atom can be conjugated with glutathione, under the action of glutathione-5 transferase.

This enzyme is characterized by a low specificity. It catalyzes the combination reactions with glutathione of aromatic, aliphatic compounds, heterocyclic radicals and aliphatic and aromatic epoxides. The ability of glutathione to form conjugates with highly reactive xenobiotic metabolites represents a high detoxification capacity.

Glutathione decreases the toxicity and mutagenic properties of metabolites. Carcinogens present in food can be classified into several groups:

a) naturally occurring substances (tryptophan, alkaloids, caffeine);

b) substances of biological pollution (alfa-toxins, from mold, corn and alkaloids). The biochemical action of alfa-toxins is explained by the fact that they are metabolized in a product that acts on chromatin by inhibiting the transcription of genes and RNA polymerase, which leads to a decrease in synthesis.

c) chemical pollution carcinogens (pesticides, HPA, nitrosamines). Endogenous synthesis of nitrosamines takes place actively in the stomach where there is a strong acidic environment conducive to nitrosamine. The process is inhibited by ascorbic acid, cysteine, reduced glutathione, glycine, asparagine, vitamin A and various antioxidants.

d) products formed by biological processing (synthetic dyes, cyclamates, saccharin, vinyl chloride). Epidemiological research has shown a positive correlation between the intake of zinc, Cd, Cu, Ca, Mg, Cr, Al, and the occurrence of cancer in the digestive tract, prostate, lung, mammary glands and blood. Research over the last decade has established a correlation between diet and immunity.

The author Dreyer believes that food status influences the immune response on several levels: • reduction of natural cellular immunity;

• reduction of antibody synthesis in deficiencies of vitamins A1, B1, B6;

• lowering the level of complement, properdin, interferon and transferrin;

• phagocytosis disorder in protein-caloric deficiency.

The importance given to diet in immunity is also highlighted by the fact that diet therapy is also given an important role in the treatment of AIDS. It should be noted that not only the deficit but also the excess food according to the mentioned ones negatively influences the immune system. Chronic infections have been found to be more common and mortality is higher in obese people, who have been shown to have reduced immunoglobulins, cellular immunity, phagocytosis and NK lymphocytes. The role of prostaglandins PGE2 is to suppress the primary and secondary immune response to the inflammatory reaction. Arachidonic acid derivation has inflammatory activity but also immunosuppressive activity because it inhibits the production of antibodies as well as cell-type immunity.

Specifically, these macrophage lipo-oxygenase pathways induce suppressor lymphocytes (TS). Aspirin and indomethacin decrease TS but increase TH and NK. The most important protective reaction that acts in the first line of

cellular defense neutralizing over 90% of the free radicals formed is the dismutation reaction which has the main advantage that it does not use the essential compounds for the cell as a substrate.

SOD 2O2 + 2H H2O + O2 catalase ----2H2 + O2 H2O + O2

The process is catabolized by the enzyme super-oxi-dismutase (SOD) considered by some researchers as the most important enzyme of aerobic life, due to the efficiency with which it achieves the neutralization of cytotoxic radicals. The hydrogen peroxide formed is broken down by catalpa into water and molecular O2, thus achieving cellular protection. Another defense system is the constant ratio of reduced glutathione, oxidized glutathione, indispensable in normal metabolism, provided by glutation-peroxidase, which contains selenium and glutathione reductase which performs the regeneration process of glucose-6-phosphate dehydrogenase dependent on NAD and NADP. The redox state of the cell expressed by the values of the NAD + and NADPH ratios is a parameter that the cell uses to balance its activity.

Free radicals resulting from energy gain, singlet oxygen is neutralized under the action of biological antioxidants in the cell. Antioxidants are those substances that inhibit the rate of oxidation by releasing H + ions, symbolically denoted by AH and which react as follows:

A * + RO2 * ------> RO2-A compound inactive

Under the influence of bio-oxidants such as tocopherols, ascorbic acid, BHT (butyl-hydroxytol), synthetic antioxidants, the regeneration of the permeability of the affected membranes takes place. Proteins and nucleic acids are the main biological substances that are protected from antioxidants. Increased oxidable lipid increases the rate of free radical formation that interacts in excess with antioxidants.

There is a wide variety of antioxidants in food (vitamin E, A, C, K, carotenes, polyphenols, amino acids and sulfur peptides). to a greater or lesser extent depending on the food. Food refining, in addition to decreasing the content of biocatalysts in food, greatly reduces the natural content of antioxidants (white flour, refined sugar, beverages). Free radicals and peroxides present in normal concentration participate in the regulation of membrane permeability, in the regulation of the growth rate of living organisms, in cell proliferation, in the regulation of membrane lipid composition, in the transmission of cellular excitation and information.

Small amounts of peroxidase are needed for ATPase to function in mitochondria. As a result, theories about free radical-induced pathologies in cardiovascular disease, cancer, and the pathologies that accompany old age are gaining ground. Increasing and decreasing the normal peroxide concentration accelerates or inhibits cell division. Imbalances in the antioxidants in lipid composition by irradiation or various pathologies can be seen as a disorder of the information transmission system. Systems for regulating cellular metabolism by oxidation reactions are found in interaction with other systems, especially nucleotides. The sensitivity of adenylate cyclase to hormones has been shown to depend on the concentration of one or another of the effector phospholipids (in the hydroxylation system).

Adenyl cyclase and phosphodiesterase are lipid-dependent enzymes. Both systems work in interactions. Therefore, acting on the cyclic nucleotide system may influence the lipid oxidation reaction and vary the rate of lipid oxidation to alter the concentration of cyclic nucleotides and thereby influence the sensitivity of cells to the action of hormones. The cell's response to hormones depends not only on cyclic nucleotides but also on the cell membrane system in general and membrane lipids in particular.

Also, the rate of antigen-antibody interaction depends on the state of the lipid phase of the membrane. The rate of lipid oxidation reaction under the action of various agents affects the lipids in all cellular organs. In the carcinogenesis, changes of the same type were observed with those of the antioxidant activity of the lipids of the mitochondria of the nucleosome of the nucleus.

Transformations of lipid micro-viscosity under the influence of adenyl-cyclase and cAMP are essential for the information transfer process in the cell that interacts between intracellular membranes in areas adjacent to the limbs. Local attachment of endoplasmic reticulum membranes to plasma and mitochondrial membranes is considered essential for the induction of lipid peroxidation in these organs. This is why obese people are more likely to get cancer from various organs infiltrated with lipids. Underweight people also get hypo-energy cancer, a level of bioenergy insufficient to repair DNA damaged by carcinogens or spontaneous mutations.

Nucleo-plasmic signals, for the induction of carcinogenesis, start from a surplus energy background in extramitochondrial ATP, cytoplasmic, predominantly anaerobic product in large quantities. Both the amount of fat

in the diet and the degree of fat saturation can influence the appearance of the tumor.

Therefore, excessive fat consumption promotes cancer by changing the hormonal profile and metabolism: cholesterol, epoxides, saturated fatty acids. Excess fat as well as excess protein can exert tumorigenic actions through metabolic products, in protein metabolism the amines formed react with nitrites forming nitrosamines with a proven carcinogenic effect. Tryptophan's metabolism also has a proven carcinogenic effect. Energy restrictions, with age, have a number of beneficial effects.

The reduction of caloric intake by 40% is also complex on the immune functions:

• decreases the circulating amount of immune complexes, increases the secretion of interleukin 2;

• the body mass decreases and the O2 requirement increases;

• DNA-RNA repair processes intensify, with changes in gene regulation and chromatin volume;

• there is a significant reduction in cytochrome oxidase and an increase in the degree of oxidation in the mitochondria of intermediates;

• inhibiting the aging of the genome and the cellular protein synthesis apparatus, decreasing the content of lipids and free radicals;

• slowing down age-related neuroendocrine changes;

• Restrictive diets reduce the oxidation of lipids in mitochondria and increase the antioxidant protection systems in the blood, the action of prolonging life is explained by the theory of free radicals.

The sub-points listed above indirectly underline the beneficial action of religious or voluntary "days of fasting" throughout a person's life. In the contemporary diet, there is a concern for the vitamin of food products and their enrichment with bio-elements and sano-genic protection factors. It has been observed that in the case of avitaminosis B1 there is a reduction in the phagocytic properties of leukocytes, a slowdown in the destruction of virulent bacteria by macrophages, a decrease in the content of complement in the blood serum.

At present, thiamine enters the complex of tuberculosis therapy and slows down the development of intoxication in the case of diphtheria. Reducing the activity of thiamine in the heart muscle leads to an attenuation of oxidative processes in the myocardium, as a result of which oxygen absorption decreases. All this causes a reduction in the level of cytoplasmic ATP which eventually manifests itself through profound morphological changes in the mitochondria.

Man, unlike most mammals, cannot synthesize vitamin C and as a result is dependent on ascorbic acid intake of foods that should not be seasonal. Ascorbic acid in food participates in the O2 transport process by increasing the activity of the cytochrome chain in cell membranes. Vitamin C in high doses activates adenyl cyclase in cell membranes and cell organs while also activating cAMP. Hypovitaminosis A is often accompanied by acute protein crisis and calorie insufficiency.

Both vitamin A and carotenoids act as donors and acceptors of electrons, participating in the transfer of electrons on either side of the cell membrane, thus influencing all stages of the Krebs cycle. Vitamin A deficiency leads to disorders of glycolysis and oxidative phosphorylation. At the same time, there is an increase in the sodium content and a decrease in the potassium content of the tissues, which affects the structure of the membrane and causes an increase in ATP-ase activity.

Vitamin A stimulates the activity of T lymphocytes, activates phagocytosis of macrophages and granulocytes, natural immunity, nonspecific anti-infective resistance. In recent years, several authors have com unique that vitamin A in doses higher than 500,000 IU / day causes an anticancer effect, as a result of stimulating the immunity of patients.

Vitamin D-rich foods play a key role in calcium metabolism, but are also important in membrane function in activating the Krebs cycle in the mitochondria. The introduction of vitamin D in the diet leads to an increase in citric acid content, especially in the kidneys, intestines, myocardium and to a lesser extent in the liver. The presence of ATP in the environment, which shows protective properties of the mitochondrial structure, has an important role for the exercise of vitamin D action in mitochondria.

Vitamins of food with tocopherols is necessary due to the fact that the refining processes of cereals and fats (the main source of vitamin E in the diet) the content of this vitamin is considerably reduced. Avitaminosis E exerts teratogenic effects. Vitamin E plays an important role in maintaining

the integrity of cell membranes and cellular organisms. Its presence in the required amount in the diet leads to an increase in the content of mitochondrial ATP and CoA in liver cells, facilitates the reactions of the Krebs cycle and oxidative phosphorylation, facilitates the transfer of thiolithic groups to the site of enzyme biosynthesis.

Tocopherols and highly active biological antioxidants have the ability to slow down the processes of lipid peroxidation in membranes, processes that cause many metabolic disorders. At the same time, it exerts a strong protective effect on the body against xenobiotics. It has been shown that the addition of alfa-tocopherols to the diet of experimental animals has a marked antimutagenic effect when administering mutagens and carcinogens, such as carbon tetrachloride. Food enrichment with as an essential role in regulating muscle and nerve activity. Ca2 + ions participate in the activation of important enzymes such as lipase, phosphatase, aconitase, etc.

At the same time, Ca2 + ions participate in the phagocytic activity of leukocytes and decrease the permeability of cell membranes to toxic substances. At the same time, Ca together with Mg performs multiple functions in the body, participating in the activity of over 50 enzymes, which transfer phosphate groups in metabolic processes and catalyze the synthesis reaction related to the breakdown of ATP and GTP. Mg2 + ions actively participate in oxidative phosphorylation by stimulating the formation of ATP from energy-rich intermediates.

It also plays an important role in the synthesis of immunoglobulins. An increased Mg deficiency can lead to lymphomas or lympho-sarcomas. Fe deficiency in diet causes two major effects; the onset of iron deficiency anemia and decreased immune capacity. Iron has an essential role in animal metabolism being a component of many enzyme systems in the respiratory chain. It intervenes in the transport of O and plays a decisive role in cellular respiration. Iron is required for the enzymatic mechanism of ribonucleotide reductase, influencing cellular DNA synthesis.

If this enzyme reduces its activity, all cellular functions are disrupted. The effect of iron deficiency on the immune response has been established in numerous studies in laboratory animals. There has been a decrease in DNA synthesis in lymphocytes, a decrease in the number of T cells, a reduction in their cytostatic activity, as well as histo-morphological and ultrastructural changes. Iron requirements are I mg / day for men and 2.8 mg / day for women. In addition to secondary risks for thyroid disease, iodine deficiency also includes the possibility of thyroid cancer.

Zinc also plays a key role in nucleic acid metabolism, protein synthesis and cell division. Fundamental subcellular research, from a plastic point of view, has shown that their membranes are made up of polyunsaturated fatty acids and most of them are represented by acids with 20-22 Ca atoms. Unsaturated fatty acids are the precursors of prostaglandins and leukotrienes, also called cellular hormones that act to regulate cAMP.

The participation of prostaglandins in the regulation of various vital processes has been established. In traditional medicine, confirmed in part by rigorous clinical research, a large number of vegetables and fruits are noted in the therapy of diseases of nutrition and metabolism. Even recent epidemiological research has shown a low incidence of cancer associated with increased consumption of garlic, and experimental research has shown a delay in the development of tumors with an increase in life after treatment with allicin, the active substance in garlic.

Numerous substances with antitumor effects have been identified in fruits and vegetables:

• introduction of enzymes that neutralize carcinogens and inhibit the enzymes responsible for inducing carcinogenesis;

• preventing healthy cell transformations into cancer cells;

• The experiments performed by Ferenezi and other authors highlighted the specific antitumor activity of beetroot, explained by the action of beta-alanine, its specific dye. It has been established that β-alanine enhances the respiration of the carcinogenic cell which is known to have a predominant anaerobic character.

Many authors explain the therapeutic action of many herbs through the effects of phenolic compounds and especially flavonoids, carotenoids, vitamin C, which activate in the cytochrome C-cytochrome oxidase system accelerating cellular respiration "in vivo" and "in vitro". Carotene is widely used in vegetable processes, especially in red, orange, green vegetables, in large quantities it is found in carrots, peppers, tomatoes, tomatoes, vegetables, peaches. β-carotene has been shown in numerous studies to be an effective cell protector and especially in inhibiting malignant processes.

Vegetables due to their high content of ß-oxidants exert a general protective effect on normal metabolism. Green vegetables and fruits are a rich source of Mg and Fe. Traditional medicine attaches great importance to germinated seeds, which are fully justified by recent biochemical research, which has

led nutritionists to expand their pharmaceuticals in germinated cereals, especially in industrialized countries.

Here we highlight the pharmaceutical product "Maza-Green", used by the Japanese and Americans as an adjunct in cancer therapy. As a result of the biosynthesis caused by the endo-zomal processes that take place during germination, vitamins B1, B2, B6 are synthesized in large quantities and there is an increase in the supply of essential amino acids available. The therapeutic action of germinated seeds can be explained by the release of free SH groups during germination.

As is known, SH groups are involved in the regulation of cellular processes having an important role in metabolic mechanisms. High reactivation of SH groups, reversible type exchange redox-thiol disulfide reflects the permanent possibilities of adapting the reaction sequences to the needs of the organism, actively integrating in the ways of producing dynamism. SH -S-S- imbalances occur during development pathological mitosis of tumor cells being involved in general malignancy.

In the aging process, there is an accumulation of the -S-S- group to the detriment of the SH group, which causes a reduction in thiol activity, a decrease in the potential for biosynthesis and self-renewal of cytoplasmic enzymes. Recently, ionic homeostasis has been given a universal role with profound implications.

Cellular ionic homeostasis influences at four levels the mechanisms of cell biosynthesis;

• on the effective action of enzymes and receptors;

• acts on the energy device;

• modulates DNA and RNA synthesis. The intake of mineral substances influences many functions of the body:

• energy exchanges (phosphorus);

• reproduction (Mg, Zn);

• hematopoiesis (Fe, Cu, Mn, Co);

• metabolism of proteins, carbohydrates, lipids. Insufficiency of these nutrients affects the body's resistance and can lead to the development of a number of diseases.

An important protective role is played by glutathione against various pollutants that attack cells: nitrites, nitrosamines, peroxides, metals and toxic substances. Glutathione oxidase neutralizes peroxides that form cytotoxic afferents by oxidizing glutathione. This enzyme combines the self-oxidizing capacity of thiols with that of selenium. Glutathione used as a substrate is the most mobile thiolic compound being present in all animal cells and easily regenerated by the pentose-phosphate shunt.

Recently, attention has been paid to the antitumor activity of lactic fermented products. Research by Kuhl and Strass has shown that the use of racemic lactic acid or yogurt (750 gr / day) has accelerated the recovery of the cancer patient. In neoplastic patients, the diet consisted of foods rich in protein but low in nucleoproteins, fresh vegetables and fruits, low in fat and was eliminated of full of sugar, sweets and alcohol. The inhibitory activity of yogurt is due to the low molecular weight compounds that are formed during lactic fermentation, compounds that can be separated by dialysis. In an urbanized society, in the conditions of industrialization, when the intake of biologically active substances is more necessary than the energy intake which in most cases is made even in excess, fruits, vegetables and especially their juices (raw cabbage juice) can play an important role as protective foods with therapeutic and sano-gene effects.

In summary, maintaining the amount of aerobic mitochondrial ATP at elevated parameters within physiological limits ensures the protection of cells against carcinogens. This can be done by:

• correct vitamins (AECB) without seasonal fluctuations;

• systematic physical activities, practiced continuously;

• elimination of refined carbohydrates from the diet and polyunsaturated fats;

• permanent maintenance of a normo-ponderal, normo-caloric status, free of physical and mental stress.

All these arguments suggest the idea that in order to prevent carcinogenesis we must ensure that almost all the cells in the body have aerobic conditions and an energy substrate corresponding to the activities carried out, [6].

CHAPTER VII

OBSERVATIONS ON THE SIGNIFICANCE OF THE ATP-MG COMPLEX IN LYMPHOCYTE WITH METABOLIC CONDITIONS

1. Observations on the significance of the ATP - Mg complex in lymphocytes of metabolic conditions

The progress of basic science has led to the proliferation of our knowledge of the mechanism of disease production and physicochemical, and biochemical conquests, with numerous applications in clinical diagnosis. Approaching the field of intracellular exploration, we asked ourselves whether the oscillations of the concentrations of cytoplasmic components around the normal range always have the significance of an "alarm phenomenon" or the detection of a risk factor.

Approaching the field of intracellular exploration, we asked ourselves whether the oscillations of the concentrations of cytoplasmic components around the normal range always have the significance of an "alarm phenomenon" or the detection of a risk factor. To answer these questions we resorted to a modern method of paraclinical investigations - luminometry - based on the study of the phenomenon of bioluminescence. By this method we studied through the luciferin-luciferase system, the production or use of lymphocytic ATP, in normal or pathological cases: allergic diseases, and malignant diseases.

Disorders of the cellular bioenergetic process can be the pathogenic basis of some pathological cellular processes. Energy-producing catabolic processes, glycolysis, cellular respiration, β-oxidation of fatty acids, and energy-consuming anabolic have a common intermediate, adenosine triphosphate (ATP).

ATP plays a major role as a reservoir, supplier, and intermediate transporter of chemical energy in living organisms, for mechanical work, metabolic processes and regulator of transmembrane ion exchange. The cytoplasmic

anaerobic glycolytic energy balance will deduce an energy gain of 2 moles of ATP for one molecule of glucose and 3 moles of ATP for one molecule of glycogen. In the anaerobic metabolism of a glucose molecule, 38 moles of ATP are formed, of which 30 moles of ATP are at the mitochondrial level in the Krebs cycle, and 8 moles at the cytoplasmic level. During the electronic transport through the respiratory chain (oxidative phosphorylation) 3 ATP bonds are formed on the transport cycle of energetic principles.

The balance of the degradation of the energetic principles can be given in the Scheme Krebs. Metabolic pathways regarding the biosynthesis of informational macromolecular components, through which genetic information is presented and transformed into proteins and nucleic acids, are correlated with the energy needs of the cell in ATP. Thc synthetic metabolic pathways of the cell are regulated by the consumption of ATP which balances the rate of functioning of cytoplasmic components at different levels and activates the corresponding enzymes. Thus, ATP remains the main source of reserve (60-70% of cellular chemical energy), for the repair processes of cytoplasmic and nuclear subfractions involved in anabolic pathways.

The homeostasis of the cell depends on the mitochondrial ATP reserve on the integrity of the respiratory chain and on the maintenance of the metabolic pathway which constantly ensures normal cell division, induction and enzymatic repression, and repression of ancestral oncogenes in chromosomes, aggressed by carcinogens. ATP is also the energy base of DNA polymerase and DNA ligase that repairs altered nucleotides in DNA under the influence of cellular aggression induced by intracellular (free radical) or extracellular (physical, chemical, and biological) toxic factors. All living cells contain ATP which is present in a fairly constant amount for each cell type and which is rapidly lost after cell death. This factor is the basis of the bioluminescence reaction by which light is measured in the enzymatic reaction of ATP degradation, catalyzed by luciferin extracted from luminescent insects (fireflies).

The amount of light produced experimentally is proportional to the amount of ATP involved in the laboratory reaction. The light reaction formula is as follows:

luciferase ATP + luciferin + O2 --> oxyluciferin + AMP + PPi + CO2 + Light

In recent years, luciferin-luciferase reagents have been specially expanded to give a constant light, effective concerning time, the light intensity is proportional to the concentration of ATP above the level of 1O-6 - 10-11 M. The method has good accuracy and reproducibility, increasing the sensitivity up to 10-12 g / ml determinant. In this study, we investigated 18 cases, including 8 clinically healthy individuals for testing for normal lymphocytic ATP levels, 6 cases of allergic patients, 2 cases of lymphocytic and chronic leukemia, a radiologically confirmed lung cancer, and a case of bone metastases with the unspecified carcinogen.

Although the number of cases is small, the error indices of the determination were excluded by using 3 typical lymphocytic ATP extraction procedures that included 3 precipitating agents for each clinical case, choosing the most accurate extract for the calculation of the amount of ATP. The ATP determinations in each case were made in a constant number of ml lymphocytes (1 x 10-6 lymphocytes/ml), regardless of the leukocyte formula of the analyzed clinical case, performing the corresponding transformations. Through these determinations, we followed the paraclinical differentiation of benign and malignant cellular metabolic conditions based on the concentration of lymphocytic ATP.

The working method was developed by the I. Cantacuzino Institute, Bucharest, based on the leaflets from the ATP putties.

Materials needed are LKB 1250 luminometer, ATP and reagent putties (TCA-EDTA), tris EDTA buffer, 4 mm LKB polystyrene tanks, and 10-500 microliter automatic micropipettes.

The main steps of the method are as follows:

1. Preparation of reagents;

2. Blood collection on heparin and I.C.-65 medium in 4 tubes;

3. Separation of lymphocytes from whole blood and their washing

3. Separation of lymphocytes from whole blood and their washing;

4. Counting lymphocytes in the Turk counting room;

5. Distribution of lymphocytes in the I.C.-65 medium at the value of 1x10-6 / cells/ml.

6. Precipitation and rupture of lymphocytes with TCA / EDTA soil. 5% 2 mM - 0.8 ml (4 ml buffer + 1 ml TCA = 5% dilution);

7. Stir the sample for 5-10 minutes at room temperature;

8. Checking cell bursts with an optical microscope;

9. Centrifugation of the sample with lysed lymphocytes;

10. Verification of the amount of supernatant protein m in the U.V. 280-260 mm (be less than 1 mg / 1 ml protein, starting at 1/50 dilution);

11. Necessary reagents are ATP Monitoring Reagent, Standard ATP, Trist EDTA Buffer 0.1 M pH 7.75, and TCA-EDTA Extractor 10% mM Solution.

The obtained results were recorded in the table and transposed graphically. Interpretation of results Mean lymphocyte ATP level for healthy clinical cases was 1.37 micromoles of ATP. In the literature, the average values have been cited in red blood cells, around 1.42 micromoles of ATP, although the metabolism of glucose is done by pentose-phosphates. The steady state of energy of the normal cell is that in which the consumption of ATP is equal to the biosynthesis of ATP. Higher ATP levels correspond to a more intense state of cell energization. We remind you that by transforming ATP - -> ADP + Pi, the free hydrolysis energy has the value of 7.30 Kcal/mol, and by transforming ATP - -> AMP + Pi, energy of 8.95 kcal/mol will be released. Given the ATP system that forms and consumes energy, the notion of energy load has been introduced with the following expression:

ADP + ATP) Se = 1/2 -- = 0.85 (AMP + ADP + ATP

For a certain value of the ATP potential, a balance is established between catabolism (glycolysis) and anabolism (gluconeogenesis). Small variations in the ATP potential on either side of the steady state are large variations in the two metabolic pathways. By increasing the ATP potential of the normal cell, the rate of glycolytic reactions decreases while the activity of enzymes in gluconeogenesis increases with the potential of ATP. However, the electric charge varies relatively little around 0.85.

If the energy load decreases below 0.85, the ATP-generating sequences are accelerated by the response of the respective regulatory components according to metabolic needs. In the case of allergic diseases, the average value determined by us is 3.69 micromoles of ATP, the highest value being recorded in the case of asthma at 4.60 micromoles of ATP. The explanation

for this much higher value than normal is the increased synthesis of ATP at the lymphocyte level in atopic terrains.

Resistance and immunity reactions in higher organisms take different forms, local and systemic, specific and nonspecific, and humoral or cellular. In most cases, several mechanisms act simultaneously, causing an immune impediment that explains the maintenance of health, sometimes even in the presence of a significant immune defect. Lymphocytes form in the body a complex network of cells capable of reacting with foreign substances, due to the presence on their surface of very specific receptors for a certain type of antigen.

The introduction of a "non-self" substance causes a series of specific interactions with certain lymphocyte subpopulations, disrupting the homeostasis of the network and triggering a series of complex phenomena such as:

• selection of cell subpopulations that carry receptors for the antigenic determinants of the respective substances.

• their numerical amplification;

• their functional differentiation and sweeping;

• activating them, etc.

The whole activity is genetically controlled and subjected to a large numberof regulatory mechanisms, which modulate the interactions of cellular constituents. Antibodies with the function of recognizing antigens do not appear as a result of the invasion of the invading antigen, but they are, as has been shown, already formed in the immune repertoire before the antigen enters the body. Regulation of IgE synthesis is dependent on T cells and involves the interaction between antigen-presenting cells with TH cells and B lymphocytes.

It has also been shown that TH and Ts lymphocytes that regulate IgE synthesis are distinct from those that influence IgG production and can be identified due to the presence of the Fc receptor for the Fc region of IgE. Regulation of IgE synthesis is mediated by a series of cellular and molecular interactions involving RFC expression on the surface of lymphoid cells. Lymphocytes exposed to high concentrations of IgE release significant amounts of regulatory factors that monitor the expression of RFC on their

surface: (GEF, glycolysis stimulating factor and GIF, glycolysis inhibiting factor).

Necessary reagents are ATP Monitoring Reagent, Standard ATP, Sad EDTA Buffer Solution 0.1 M pH 7.75, and TCA-EDTA Extractor 10% mM Solution. The obtained results were recorded in the table and transposed graphically. Interpretation of results

The mean lymphocyte ATP level for healthy clinical cases was 1.37 micromoles of ATP. In the literature, the average values have been cited in red blood cells, around 1.42 micromoles of ATP, although the metabolism of glucose is done by pentose-phosphates. The steady state of energy of the normal cell is that in which the consumption of ATP is equal to the biosynthesis of ATP. Higher ATP levels correspond to a more intense state of cell energization. We remind you that by transforming ATP - -> ADP + Pi, the free hydrolysis energy has the value of 7.30 Kcal/mol, and by transforming ATP - -> AMP + Pi, energy of 8.95 kcal/mol will be released. Given the ATP system that forms and consumes energy, the notion of energy load has been introduced with the following expression:

ADP + ATP) Se = 1/2 - = 0.85 (AMP + ADP + ATP

For a certain value of the ATP potential, a balance is established between catabolism (glycolysis) and anabolism (gluconeogenesis). Small variations in the ATP potential on either side of the steady state are large variations in the two metabolic pathways. By increasing the ATP potential of the normal cell, the rate of glycolytic reactions decreases while the activity of enzymes in gluconeogenesis increases with the potential of ATP. However, the electric charge varies relatively little around 0.85.

If the energy load decreases below 0.85, the ATP-generating sequences are accelerated by the response of the respective regulatory components according to metabolic needs. In the case of allergic diseases, the average value determined by us is 3.69 micromoles of ATP, the highest value being recorded in the case of asthma at 4.60 micromoles of ATP. The explanation for this much higher value than normal is the increased synthesis of ATP at the lymphocyte level in atopic terrains.

Resistance and immunity reactions in higher organisms take different forms, local and systemic, specific and nonspecific, and humoral or cellular. In most cases, some mechanisms act simultaneously, causing an immune impediment that explains the maintenance of health, sometimes even in the presence of a significant immune defect. Lymphocytes form in the body a

complex network of cells capable of reacting with foreign substances, due to thepresence on their surface of very specific receptors for a certain type of antigen.

The introduction of a "non-self" substance causes a series of specific interactions with certain lymphocyte subpopulations, disrupting the homeostasis of the network and triggering a series of complex phenomena such as: • selection of cell subpopulations that carry receptors for the antigenic determinants of the respective substances; • their numerical amplification; • their functional differentiation and sweeping; • activating them, etc. The whole activity is genetically controlled and subjected to a large number of regulatory mechanisms, which modulate the interactions of cellular constituents.

Antibodies with the function of recognizing antigens do not appear as a result of the invasion of the invading antigen, but they are, as has been shown, already formed in the immune repertoire before the antigen enters the body. Regulation of IgE synthesis is dependent on T cells and involves the interaction between antigen-presenting cells with TH cells and B lymphocytes. It has also been shown that TH and Ts lymphocytes that regulate IgE synthesis are distinct from those that influence IgG production and can be identified due to the presence of the Fc receptor for the Fc region of IgE. Regulation of IgE synthesis is mediated by a series of cellular and molecular interactions involving RFC expression on the surface of lymphoid cells.

Lymphocytes exposed to high concentrations of IgE release significant amounts of regulatory factors that monitor the expression of RFC on their surface: (GEF, glycolysis stimulating factor and GIF, glycolysis inhibiting factor).

The complex biochemical study of target cell activation showed that stimulation of cellular receptors with externally active pharmacological agents initiates a chain of biochemical reactions with a final intracellular effect. According to some researchers, ATPase normally competes with an adenylate cyclase for ATP, resulting in the direct formation of inactivated AMP without the formation of active cAMP. Stimulation of adenyl cyclase with sympathomimetics would allow the direct use of ATP to increase cAMP.

In the presence of Ca and Mg, cAMP controls the activity of enzymes, cells, and permeability barriers normally to stimulate cell synthesis and secretion. CAMP also regulates antibody synthesis in B lymphocytes, slows the rate of cell division, inhibits ARM synthesis, and slows down protein synthesis. In the malignant cell, cAMP has lower concentrations than in the normal cell. In anaphylactic reactions, the role of cAMP is exactly the opposite as in other "second messenger" secretory systems.

Like language with limited vocabulary, the immune system has a basic lexicon, represented by genetic information encoded in germ genes in germ cells. The "generative capacity" of the immune system has been demonstrated experimentally, externalized by the possibility of mutational events in proliferative B cells. It allows the formation of antibodies with valid regions other than those encoded by the stem cells from which the B cell precursors were formed. Also, the immune system is mainly oriented towards the internal environment, specific to the body to which it belongs (self-centred).

Due to this behavior, it produces anti-idiotypic antibodies to its antibodies that accidentally disrupt the dynamic harmony of the system. Allergic tissue damage usually involves the active participation of several categories of monocyte cells, neutrophils, and basophils, without excluding the intervention of platelets. In the immune system, the initial process of phagocytosis is associated with the onset of a respiratory burst corresponding to the activation of latent metabolic pathways in neutrophils.

The "respiratory cascade" has four phases, the existence of which has been demonstrated by metabolic inhibitors:

1. Immediate increase in O2 and ATP consumption;

2. Increased oxidation of glucose by the shunt-hexozo-mono-phosphates (SHMP);

3. Enzymatic stimulation of NADH- and NADPH-oxidases and production of superoxide (O2_) radicals.

4. Production of H2O2 and unstable intermediates, such as hydroxyl (OH) and singlet oxygen (O2) radicals.

During this phase, the chemotactic factors stimulate the aerobic metabolism of granulocytes by 25-125% and the SHMP activity by 100-600%. T lymphocytes sensitized after first contact with the antigen also amplify their metabolic status compared to non-desensitized lymphocytes, not specific to

the antigen. In the peripheral blood 60-80% of the lymphocyte populations are represented by T lymphocytes, and 25-30% by B lymphocytes.

By phenotypic criteria, mature T cell subpopulations were grouped into two broad, functionally distinct categories: 1. Cells with adjustment functions: T helper (TH), T amplifier (Ta) and T suppressor (Ts). 2. Cells with effector functions: cytotoxic T (Tc) and TDH cells with a role in hypersensitivity phenomena. Normal-positive and neoplastic B cells have the ability to "present" T cell antigens.

This "presentation" by nonspecific B cells is subject to the same rules as for macrophages and other antigen-presenting cells. In allergic processes, increasing the concentration of ATP and increasing the concentration of cAMP in mast cells inhibits the release of mediators such as vasoactive amines, opposing aggressions at a threshold level on atopic terrain in asymptomatic conditions or clinical calm. Under these conditions, the level of ATP will be constantly increased.

In this way, it is necessary to observe that the determination of lymphocyte ATP could be used in the detection of atopic lands and allergic conditions. To verify these observations, the study was resumed on a new lot of patients mathematically processing the data in the table with methods adapted according to the number of investigated cases.

Regarding the study of malignancies, we note the values: 4.30 - 4.55 micromoles of ATP for chronic lymphocytic leukemia and 3.20 - 3.65 micromoles of ATP for lung cancer and bone metastases, respectively. The explanation of the high values in these cases is complex. The literature records values of 3.32 micromoles of ATP in tumor cells obtained by biochemical dosing. In the cancer cell, glycolysis goes beyond benign tumors and cellular hypercatabolic conditions.

An important aspect of glycolysis in the tumor cell can be considered the fact that the functional differences of ATP formed on the one hand from glycolysis and on the other hand from respiration have certain relations with the special properties of the tumor cell. Warburg designated glycolysis ATP as inferior morphologically, assuming that intramitochondrial and structurally fixed ATP, which occurred following the Krebs cycle coupled with oxidative phosphorylation, is capable of acting with differential synthesis by normal metabolic pathways. ATP - glycolytic from the cancerous tumor cell, whose production is intensified 30 times more than the production of ATP from normal glycolysis in the unstructured

fundamental plasma of the cell can migrate by diffusion inside the cytoplasm.

The cell nucleus, capable only of a limited proportion of its energy, can more easily obtain it from this free ATP which is more mobile than oxidative mitochondrial ATP. This captured ATP provides the energy needed for nucleic acids and proteins as well as the processes of chromosome movement during cell mitosis. ATP from glycolysis may promote the processes of intracytoplasmic movement that occur during cell division. Cellular respiration is related to malignancy, in the sense that intense glycolysis and malignancy would be associated with lower respiration and relative benignity and hypercatabolic conditions, with lower than malignant glycolysis and considerably increased oxidation.

Therefore, in the prevention of carcinogenesis, it is recommended to intensify the flow of electrons at the mitochondrial level, increasing the level of mitochondrial ATP by supplementing non-enzymatic electron transporters (ascorbic acid, glutathione), vitamins without seasonal fluctuations (vitamin A, B, C, E), consumption of vegetables and raw foods rich in antioxidants (ß-alanine retinoids, vegetable polyphenols), disconnecting the body from daily stresses that establish the predominance of anaerobic metabolism. If lymphocytic ATP in chronic lymphocytic leukemia is increased by more than 4 micromoles of ATP as an expression of increased cellular metabolism due to abnormal divisions in the process of malignant multiplication, ATP in lung cancer as in metastases is increased by more than 3μM by a systemic effect, lymphatic system aggressively or without the aggression of tumor antigens.

Also, determining ATP levels above 3 micromoles can be a warning sign of a malignant disease if they occur against the metabolic background of the chronic consumptive disease. I emphasize that if the concentration of glycolytic ATP in the cancer cell is very high due to the high synthesis of DNA and protons, in the cancerous lymphocytes, the glycolytic ATP is raised too high parameters due to their intense activation by malignant cells by direct contact. and signs of the biofield, being ready to destroy them, stopped at this stage of waiting by numerous barriers that oppose them.

The cells that carry the immunological specificity and whose reaction with the antigen determines the cellular response characteristic of delayed hypersensitivity belong to a special population represented by TDH lymphocytes. Activated TDH cells synthesize and secrete a large number of lymphocytes and transfer factors. They are essential in the recruitment of

other types of circulating cells, with effector swarm, directly in hypersensitivity: Tc, NK and K lymphocytes.

By being able to be present and active cytotoxically without prior immunization, NK cells can recognize tumor cells very early in their development and perform their role of "surveillance" through the quality of effector cells. K cells (Killer Cells) have antibody-dependent activity. They are stimulated by interferons and interleukin-2. This property may have important therapeutic applications in the future, by expanding its role in the body's resistance to tumors.

They use "non-safe" cells and sometimes counteract the early removal of the first malignant cells, through immunological "surveillance". A killer T cell can act successively on several target cells either directly or with the participation of complement or other effector cells. Their activated state is expressed by an increased metabolic state in ATP. Experimenting on isolated mitochondria, German researchers found in malignant cells a deficiency of mitochondrial ATP 3-40% of normal value, this deficiency being compensated in the cytoplasm by glycolytic ATP. In this way, ATP in diseased tissue cells becomes a functional marker for malignant disease. The engine of malignancy is undoubtedly mostly in the malignant cell itself.

From this point of view, cancer must be seen primarily as a cellular phenomenon, because malignant cell biosynthesis takes place with the consumption of energy generally from the macro-ergic bonds of ATP stored in excess in the cytoplasm. I emphasize the following catabolic observations by enhancing cellular respiration. During the metabolic, physiological resting state, there is a normalization of the ATP content to values between 1-1.52 micromoles, the macro-energic compound favoring the development of the synthesis process and the restoration of the normal capacity of the cell.

• If the cellular excitation is taken to physiological extremes, as in benign hypercatabolic states, there is an increase in the amount of ATP (> 2.75 micromoles), which increases the activity of enzymes.

In malignant metabolic states, the cellular ATP content increases by more than 3 micromoles by intensifying anaerobic and aerobic glycolysis with decoupling of oxidative phosphorylation, increasing the rate of renewal of proteins, then RNA-DNA and phospholipids. In future investigations, I will try to open up the prospects for an early diagnosis of malignancies as well

as a strategy for monitoring treatments by determining lymphocytic ATP, especially in leukemic diseases.

Also is considered the possibility of modulating cellular bioenergy by using inhibitors of cytoplasmic glycolysis (fluorine derivatives) with specific tropism for tumor tissue. Determinations of ATP concentrations by luminometry can be successfully extended to subjects with acquired or inherited cellular disorders, such as enzymatic deficiencies (pyruvate kinase, hexokinase or glucose-phosphate dehydrogenase), hemolytic conditions, qualitative disorders of platelets, acute tumors, and tumors. myeloproliferative, leukemoid reactions, AIDS. We further reproduce the actual work technique as well as the percentage notes involved in the reaction times.

Working technique

Preparation of reagents > ATP Monitoring reagent - fill the lyophylised contents of the vial with 5 ml of distilled water. This will allow the testing of 50 samples using a 0.1 ml reagent volume with a 0.9 ml sample volume, resulting in a total reagent volume of 1 ml. > Standard ATP - make up to 10 ml with distilled water. This will give a 1 x 106 M ATP solution.

- It is recommended that the standard ATP solution be prepared for only a few days. > Tris EDTA, solution buffer - dilute with distilled water (pH titrated with acetic acid), 500 ml. This solution can be used for sample dilution. > TCA-EDTA, solution 10%, 4 millimoles - dilute with 100 1 of distilled water. This solution can be stored in the refrigerator for several months. General procedure: all samples should have a volume of 0.9 ml in addition to 0.1 ml of ATP Monitoring reagent solution, added at the beginning of the test. All sample dilutions will be made in 0.1 M tris acetate, 2 mM EDTA pH 7.75, written on the vial.

Separation of lymphocytes from whole blood on a fig gradient 10 ml of blood is collected on Heparin 100 units of H / ml of blood + 3 ml of IC-65 medium in 4 tubes.

• Prepare IC 65 separation medium, 9%, in distilled water and Oditson 34% in distilled water; mix 24 parts with 10 parts Odiston.

• Insert 3 ml of mixture into the centrifuge tank.

• Carefully insert 3-5 ml of whole blood on the separating medium on the wall of the test tube.

• Centrifuge for 20 minutes at 2000 rpm.

• In the centrifuge tanks will be obtained: at the surface, in the plasma ring in medium, a ring of lymphocytes and macrophages, below is the Phicol and Oditson medium, and to the base of the tank is sediment, macrophage, polynuclear red blood cells and dead cells.

The lymphocyte ring is carefully removed with a Pasteur pipe.

• Place in 25 ml cuvettes, 3 ml IC 65 medium and lymphocyte ring to wash the lymphocytes.

• Wash 3 times every 10 minutes at 1500 rpm and twice 10 minutes at 1000 rpm (the first wash removes the ficol-edition environment from the Turkish chamber).

• Resuspend the washed lymphocytes m 10 m and medium IC 65 + 0.2 ml 2% calf serum.

• After resuspension, the suspension is placed in Jena glass Petri dishes, previously stored at 36 ° C.

• Leave on the thermostat for 30 °, 30 minutes for the macrophages to adhere to the glass.

• Lymphocytes are counted again after macrophages join the Turkish chamber. • Wash the lymphocytes 3 times in 3 ml medium I IC 65 in 25 ml cuvettes.

• Distribute in IC 65 the required amount of lymphocytes per ml (1 x 10 cells/ml). • If the lymphocytes are increased, to more than one million / ml, we will dilute the sample, and if the lymphocytes are lower than one million / ml, we resuspend, wash and centrifuge them so that we can calculate them at 1 x 1O6 cells/ml. • Lysis of lymphocytes with an extractant (TCA / EDTA sol.% 4 mM). 3. The technique of counting lymphocytes in the Turkish chamber.

• Mix well the suspension to be counted.

• Take 0.2 ml of the suspension and place it in a well containing 0.2 ml of eosin.

• Mix well with a Pasteur pipette. • Insert a glass capillary into the mixture.

• Insert the capillary suspension into the counting chamber, taking care to fill the chamber. The dilution is taken into account when calculating the number of cells/ml. a) The actual measurement of ATP • 200 microliters ATP Monitoring reagent with 600 microliters acetate buffer, prepared according to the above model, is introduced with the micropipettes into the luminometer tank.

• The background LKB is measured on the luminometer, light emission in mV, noting the value of B (mV).

• Then add 200 microliters of the sample to that dilution.

• Measure the constant level of light emission on the luminometer screen, noting the value of S1 (mV), (20-30 "), during which time several readings of the same sample will be repeated and the lowest values will be noted. of S1.

• 10 microliters of standard ATP (I1) are then added to the cuvettes. The highest values of I1 will be noted, depending on them, obtaining the level of ATP at the highest amount of TCA used. S1 (mV) - B1 (mV) ATP (micromoles) = x 10 uM ATP st. I1 (mV).

Procedural notes:

• The optimal pH for the luminescence reaction is 7.75, its verification is done at 1/50 dilution. Anions inhibit the reaction in the following ascending order: chlorine, bromine, nitrogen, and iodine. To do this, they must be removed from the environment. The inclusion of EDTA in the extract medium makes the inactivation of ATP conversion enzymes irreversible, therefore, if possible, EDTA should be included in any relationship with ATP.

• The sample should be mixed with an equal volume of 10% TCA / EDTA ice, -4% mM. To obtain concentrations of standard ATP other than the present one, we will make dilutions with tris RDTA buffer. Composition tris EDTA buffer, the solution required for dilution ATP Monitoring reagent: 6.060 gr. tris + 0.372 gr. EDTA; dilute with distilled water to pH 7.75, 600 ml. This buffer can also be used for sample dilution. Extractors that can be used:

• TCA / EDTA solution 10%, 4 mM required for sample volume: 10 gr. Tricloracetic acid + 0.144 gr. EDTA; dilute with 100 ml of distilled water. This solution can be stored in the refrigerator for several months.

• Triton X-100 EDTA 2% mM solution; 0.2 triton X + 0.144 EDTA; dilute with 100 gr. distilled water. All samples should be 0.9 ml to which 0.1 ml of ATP Monitoring reagent solution should be added at the beginning of the test. All sample dilutions will be made in 0.1 M tris acetate 2 mM EDTA (pH 7.75).

Before completing the test, make dilutions greater than 1/50 to check the amount of protein. We can make progressive dilutions of TCA: 1-2.5 - 5% in 2 mM EDTA for each sample and check under the light microscope what concentration will complete the best lysis of lymphocytes.

Lymphocyte lysis is done by mixing 0.9 ml sample (1 x 10 6 lymphocytes resuspended in 0.1 M tris acetate) with TCA sol. 1-2.5-5-10% 4 mM, in equal amounts (V / V) which we will mix (0.8 ml) mechanically for 5-10 minutes at room temperature, after which we will check the lysis under a microscope. If we perform lysis with triton X 100, we will also make a mixture with the V / V sample. In the present work, the determinations were made by lysing the lymphocytes with 0.8 ml 5% TCA in 2 mM EDTA.

For normal cases the average value of the background was 13.12mV; for S1 the average values of around 197.15 mV were registered and for I1 the average value of 1534 mV. Through the luminometric method, the disease state considered as a deficit or bioenergetic surplus of the organism finds new perspectives of diagnosis and prognosis,

Chapter quick Significance of ATP - Mg Complex in Endocrine Regulation Hormones are endogenous biochemical effectors secreted directly into the blood by specialized cells of the endocrine glands in the endocrine system or by endocrine cells in individualized anatomical structures. Transported by blood to the target effector organs, they exert a stimulating, integrating action on physiological and metabolic or inhibitory processes. In target cells, hormones act on two main mechanisms:

1. Activation or inhibition of enzymes by cyclic AMP or cyclic GMP; 2. Genetically controlled enzymatic induction or repression. Many non-steroidal hormones, such as adrenaline, glucagon, and other polypeptide hormones, exert their action very rapidly (30-60 ") by binding to specific receptors on the target cell membrane and thereby activating the enzyme adenyl cyclase. protein kinase.

2. Adenyl cyclase catalyzes the conversion of ATP to cyclic AMP. CAMP can activate, through proteinase, ATP-dependent enzyme systems, which can influence cell membrane permeability and, as such, cellular

transformations. Active cAMP in cells is converted to inactive AMP under the action of an enzyme called phosphodiesterase.

Adenyl-cyclase phosphodiesterase enzyme catalyzes follow reaction:

ATP -> AMP-c --> AMP.
Mg adenyl-cyclase- Hormone --> Membrane receptor --> ATP -> c-AMP + p protein kinase
Hormone --> Membrane receptor ----> ATP ----> ADP + p-protein

Among the complete non-steroidal hormones, insulin is of particular importance in intermediate metabolism. Insulin exerts a metabolic action based on its ability to function as a cyclic anti-AMP factor. In organs sensitive to the action of insulin, it increases the permeability of the cell wall for monosaccharides, amino acids, and fatty acids, thus increasing their cytoplasmic concentration and the possibility of metabolism (adipose tissue, liver, and muscle).

Insulin induces the biosynthesis of key glycolysis enzymes: hexokinase, phosphofructokinase, and phospho-enol-pyruvate-kinase. This activates both glycolysis and the Krebs cycle. Under the influence of insulin, the degradation of glucose by the pentose-phosphates is increased, through which important amounts of NADPH2 are formed. Insulin stimulates the biosynthesis of found acids as well as fats in general.

The effect of insulin on protein metabolism is to stimulate protein biosynthesis due to increased penetration of amino acids into cells as well as increased RNA synthesis in cells with specific receptors. Through its mitochondrial action, insulin intervenes directly in the ATP-AMP relationship and conditions the coupling of tissue respiration with oxidative phosphorylation.

Highlighting its action on mitochondrial contraction, through experimental work, altering its cycle in diabetes, highlights the integration of the above assumptions in the molecular theory of insulin. It has been found that in experimental diabetes there is an alteration of the swelling-contraction cycle of the mitochondria.

The described effect is found in hepatic muscle mitochondria in normal cells, where ATP-induced mitochondrial contraction in the presence of insulin is greater than ATP-induced contraction in the presence of cysteine. Glucagon is the hormone antagonist of insulin and acts on the target organs,

especially the liver and adipose tissue via the cAMP-adenylate-cyclase system.

The parathyroid hormone, parathyroid hormone, mobilizes Ca2 + and P2 + from the bones, induces inhibition of osteoblasts and stimulation of osteoclast activity. Ca and P mobility in the bone can be explained by the influence that the parathyroid hormone exerts on glycolysis and the Krebs cycle in osteoclasts.

These phenomena lead to the accumulation of citric acid and other organic acids that chelate Ca from the bones, thus favoring its mobilization. Parathyroid hormone is involved in mitochondrial cellular respiration and active transport of Ca in the mitochondria. Calcitonin inhibits osteoclast activation and stimulates osteoblast activation and thus Ca and P deposits in the bone system. Stimulation of bone mineralization causes a decrease in the blood concentration of Ca and P. Thymus hormones (thymic, thymine, thyme-pectin I and II) stimulate the proliferation of lymphoid cells and the differentiation of T lymphocytes, thus intervening in the body's immune processes

Erythro0poetine accelerates the formation and maturation of erythrocytes, especially in hypoxic conditions. Prostaglandins are derived from fatty acids with 20 carbon atoms that may have 3.4 or 5 C = C double bonds in the molecule. The most common precursor of Prostaglandins is a widespread arachidonic acid in tissues. Under the influence of cyclooxygenase, it is converted to a cyclic endoperoxide (PGG2), the immediate precursor of prostaglandins, thromboxane and prostacyclin.

Prostaglandins act on both adenyl-cyclase and guanyl cyclase, influencing the synthesis of cAMP and cGMP. Through these secondary messengers, prostaglandins influence the secretion of endocrine glands such as the thyroid, adrenal glands, and parathyroid glands. Excitation or damage to cell membranes also triggers prostaglandin biosynthesis by releasing unsaturated fatty acids from phospholipids, which results in active stimulation of neighbor cells in the same tissue or tissues.

Other hormones such as bradykinin, acetylcholine, and histamine, also stimulate prostaglandin synthesis. Prostaglandins are involved in inflammatory processes and some non-steroidal anti-inflammatory drugs (aspirin, indomethacin) justify, at least in part, their pharmacodynamic action on their ability to inhibit prostaglandin biosynthesis. Thyroid

hormones are derived from the amino acids thyroxine (thyroxine, T4), and tri-iodothyronine (T3).

Thyroid hormones exert multiple effects in the body to ensure the regulation, integration and coordination of the main physiological functions of the body.

Their somatotropic action is due to the role of thyroid hormones in the biosynthesis and distribution of structural and enzymatic proteins as well as nucleic acids. It creates a hypercatabolic state. At even higher concentrations, thyroid hormones cause the decoupling of oxidative phosphorylation with a decrease in respiratory rate (P / O).

Mitochondrial oxidation reductions are also activated because thyroid hormones cause changes in the permeability of mitochondrial membranes that lead to mitochondrial ballooning. Low hormone levels also lead to a decoupling of phosphorylation with disruption of aerobic metabolism. Therefore, cancer may be due to hypofunction or glandular hyperfunction that creates intracellular metabolic conditions for the expression of chromosomal oncogenes.

Through the hormones mentioned and with a large number of enzyme systems, which they influence, the thyroid hormones control the entire intermediate metabolism. Catecholamine biosynthesis occurs in the mitochondria of chromaffin cells in the adrenal medulla and the mitochondria of peripheral and central neurons when L-tyrosine is transformed into dopamine.

The physiological role of catecholamines is based on their stimulatory action on adrenergic receptors. The metabolic action of adrenaline is exerted through receptors that are associated with adenyl cyclase on the target cell membrane. By stimulating the cAMP system, adenyl cyclase influences carbohydrate metabolism, intensifying it in the opposite direction to the action of insulin, adrenaline being the most active natural antagonist of insulin.

Thus, adrenaline has a global hyperglycemic effect because it accentuates phosphorylation, activating phosphorylase-b-kinase. This enzyme catalyzes the conversion of phosphorylase "b" to more active phosphorylase "a".
phosphorylase b 2 phosphorylase b + 4 ATP ---phosphorylase a + 4 ADP
kinases

Under the action of phosphorylase "a" glycogen cleaves to form glucose-1-P, which in the liver and muscles oxidizes intensely to CO_2 and H_2O, leading to a calorific effect. Noradrenaline does not influence phosphorylase "b". Both catecholamines cause an increase in lipolysis in adipose tissue via cAMP.

Due to their glycogenolytic, lipolytic, and calorigenic effects, the global activation of catecholamines is catabolizing. The main biochemical mechanism by which catecholamines act, in their capacity as activators of b adrenergic receptors, is to increase the biosynthesis of cAMP, a process in which ATP, GTP and possibly other organ or tissue-dependent factors participate. Steroid hormones. Structurally, it is derived from the so-called C_7H_{28} hydrocarbon also known as strain, (cyclo-pentane-perhydro-phenanthrene).

Hormones secreted by the endocrine glands are taken up by plasma receptors that carry them to target organs and cells. nuclear receptors and intervene especially in the transcription of the genetic message. This stimulates the synthesis of proteins and especially of specific enzymes whose formation forms the basis of the physiological action of steroid hormones.

After steroid hormones exert their biological action in their cells, their catabolism takes place for excretion, with the participation of the redox chain leading to the appearance of hydroxylated compounds. Estrogen hormones (estrone, estriol, estradiol) control the synthesis of structural and functional proteins at the transcription of the genetic message in the uterine lining.

Progestin hormones influence the structure of the vaginal mucosa, the development of mammary glands and glandular acini by the same molecular mechanism. An increase in progesterone in the blood causes a direct or long-term decrease in either the hypothalamus, FSH and LH secretion through a short or long feedback process.

Testosterone, the male sex hormone itself, secreted by the testicle and in small amounts by the adrenal cortex and ovary, is transported to the target organs by blood bound to a specific transport protein. In target cells, under the action of a 5th testosterone reductase enzyme, testosterone is reduced to the 5th α dihydroxy-testosterone, the active form. The main mechanism by which it plays its complex physiological role is to regulate and control the synthesis of structural and functional proteins in the transcription of the

genetic message from DNA to RNA.

Testosterone can also influence the permeability of cell membranes as well as the activity of some enzymes through allosteric mechanisms. The anabolic effect of sex hormones is explained by their influence on protein metabolism with increasing muscle mass with muscle hypertrophy. We emphasize the participation of testosterone in the lymphocyte system in the sense of physiological stimulation of helper T cells.

Adrenal corticoid hormones have glucocorticoid function, mineralocorticoid function and sex hormone function. Like all steroid hormones, corticosteroid hormones exert their action inside the target organs, influencing the biosynthesis of DNA-dependent proteins.

The hypothalamic-pituitary-adrenal cortex axis is the main mechanism that ensures the adaptation of homeostasis, the balance of the body concerning all environmental factors. Corticosteroids intervene in the adaptation to environmental hazards and overloads. Cortisol and hormones with glucocorticoid action strongly influence carbohydrate metabolism, and stimulate glycogenesis by inhaling phosphorylation and activating glycogen synthesis. They influence gluconeogenesis by activating some enzymes.

They influence gluconeogenesis by activating some enzymesIt influences gluconeogenesis by activating some enzymes with an important role in gluconeogenesis, such as pyruvate carboxylase, phosphoenolpyruvate carboxylase, fructose 1-6 bi-phosphatase, glucose-6-phosphatase.

It also exerts a hyperglycemic action on protein metabolism, with cortisol acting differently, stimulating the biosynthesis of enzymatic proteins and the liver and inhibiting them in peripheral organs and tissues. In lipid metabolism, glucocorticoids intervene by exerting a global lipolytic action.

Aldosterone influences mineral metabolism, and so the exchange of Na-K, producing activation of the sodium pump. The complex biological and especially anti-inflammatory and immunosuppressive action of glucocorticoids, as cell membrane stabilizers and especially stimulators of suppressor T cells, increases in parallel with the induced cAMP concentration, due to the ACTH action on the adrenal cortex. Based on some mechanisms, corticosteroids influence the carbohydrate, lipid, protein, and mineral metabolism, regulating the activity of devices and systems. Steroidogenesis has been shown to increase in parallel with the intracellular concentration of cAMP. It is accepted that the stage influenced by cAMP in the adrenal gland is that of converting cholesterol to pregnenolone.

There is evidence that some actions of prostaglandins, calcitonin, and insulin, are also manifested through cAMP, the hormones mentioned also acting on adenyl cyclase or phospho-di-esterase, (usually by replacing it). The highest and most complex level of regulation and control of physiological and metabolic processes in the body is the central nervous system and the vegetative system.

Across the entire nervous system, acetyl-coline plays the role of a typical neurotransmitter. Acetylcholine, in the nerve cell, is synthesized from choline and acetyl CoA. under the action of cholinesterase with the participation of ATP.

ATP-ase-Choline + Acetyl CoA -Acetylcholine ATP ---> AMP + P-P

Nerve tissue is endowed with enzymatic equipment necessary for the metabolic processes that take place at this level: carbohydrate and lipid metabolism. It also contains respiratory chain enzymes. Maintaining nerve activity requires a permanent supply of energy, provided by

ATPase, an enzyme that breaks down one of the macro-energetic bonds in ATP. Through the action of ATPase, energy is also released in the synthesis processes of acetylcholine and glutamine.

Without claiming to deplete the full range of neurosecretory, glandular or tissue hormones, in this chapter I wanted to highlight the implications of certain hormones in cell catabolism or anabolism. In conclusion, I emphasize that hormonal regulation takes place in hierarchically organized themes, and at the highest level is the nervous system which through endorphins and hypothalamic bodies controls the activity of the pituitary gland in terms of somatotropic, endo-corticotropic, melano-tropic and anti-diuresis.

Also, the endocrine gland, the epiphysis, through the endocrine cells regulates the activity of the endocrine glands and influences the functions of the effector organs, by directly or indirectly, positively or negatively, controlling the enzymatic reactions that take place inside the cells of the tissue and organs.

On the other hand, through a self-regulating feedback mechanism, the concentration of products resulting in a metabolic stage can positively or negatively influence the development of processes at higher regulatory levels, [7].

2. Variable levels of conserved energy of APT in malignant hematologic and nonhematologic malignant disease

Chronic lymphocytic leukemia, (also known as "chronic lymphoid leukemia" or CLL), is a type of leukemia or cancer of the white blood cells, and lymphocytes. The cells accumulate mainly in the bone marrow and blood. Morphologically, these cells resemble mature lymphocytes in the peripheral blood. In the majority of patients with chronic CLL, the cells are clonal B cells arrested in the B-cell differentiation pathway between pre-B cells and mature B cells. Only 2-5% of patients with chronic CLL exhibit a T-cell phenotype. In CLL the DNA of a B cell is mutated so that it can't fight infection, but it grows out of control and crowds out the healthy blood cells that can fight infection.

Theoretical studies have suggested that elevated concentrations of adenosine triphosphate (ATP) in malignant B cell lymphocytes from CLL impair the P53 gene to induce apoptosis of cells.

Apoptosis is regulated by a cascade of proteins called caspases that are present in all cell forms as pro-form. After cleavage, caspases become active and initiate pathways leading to apoptosis. The pro-apoptotic proteins Bax, Bad, Bak and Bid induce programmed cell death. Death resistance of hypoxia takes place on at least two levels, within mitochondria and the cytosol.

Accumulation of Bax in the mitochondria causes the release of cytochrome C in the cytosol which is strongly reduced under hypoxic environment conditions. Apoptosis, performed within the extrinsic pathway, is initiated by death ligands, such as Fas ligand or tumor necrosis factor (TNF), which ultimately leads to the activation of caspases 8 and the activation of apoptosis protein activating factor (APAF). All hematopoietic cells, especially lymphoid cells, express Bcl-2, mainly in the nucleus and endoplasm reticulum. The oncogene Bcl-2 may be a general suppressor of genes that directly regulate apoptosis. This action can be inhibited by apoptosis drugs, such as Venetoclax, **[Scheme 6].**

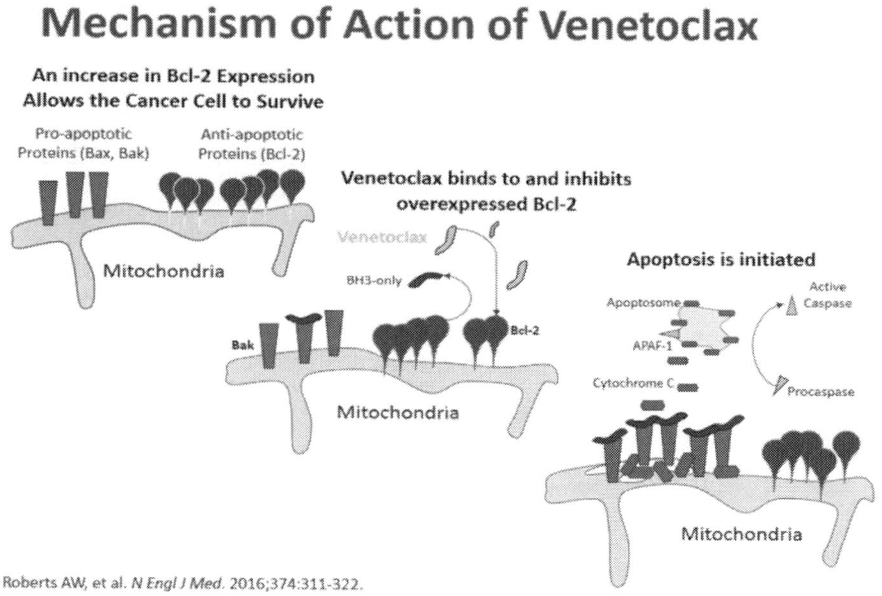

Scheme 6: Action mechanism of Venetoclax drug by inhibition of Bcl-2 oncogene in malignant lymphoproliferative diseases

The main objective of the study was to measure the intracellular ATP concentrations in B lymphocytes from patients with CLL, and compare to ATP concentrations in B and T cells from healthy patients and patients with other malignant diseases or non-malignant disease.

The main objective of the study was to measure the intracellular ATP concentrations in B lymphocytes from patients with CLL and compare them to ATP concentrations in B and T cells from healthy patients and patients with other malignant diseases or non-malignant diseases.

The measurement of ATP was made by the standard principle of bioluminescence on automatic analyzer LKB, using ATP monitoring reagent, ATP Standard, (10^6 Mol ATP/ ml), buffer solution Tris-EDTA, TCA-EDTA lyse. All results were statistically analyzed by Excel program. T lymphocytes were obtained from the peripheral blood of healthy individuals

and hospitalized patients with selected diseases from the departments of Internal Medicine and Oncology. The patient cohort was a total of 75 patients (50 males and 25 females) consisting of the following groups were examined: 25 patients (mean ages 55 ± 0.5)), with allergic diseases (allergic rhinitis, allergic dermatitis, chronic allergic asthma), 25 patients(mean ages 58 ± 1.8) with non-hematopoietic malignant diseases (lung cancer, bone metastasis) and 25 patients with confirmed hematopoietic malignant disorders, in the diagnosis of CLL In addition, 120 blood samples from apparently healthy donors (mean ages 40.02 ±12.01) were also examined. The May Grunwald-Giemsa method was used to determine the microscopic appearance of peripheral blood lymphocytes from patients with incipient CLL disease, who had not had any treatment or hematopoietic stem cell transplantation (HSCT). Morphologically, the cells resembled normal mature clonal B cells arrested in the B- cell differentiation pathway intermediate between pre-B cells and mature B cells lymphocytes although slightly larger, and more fragile when smeared onto a glass slide (smudge cells). Lymphocytes were separated from peripheral blood by centrifugation in a Ficoll gradient for 20 minutes at 2000 rcf / minute.

Lysis of lymphocytes with TCA-EDTA was performed after cell counts were adjusted to 1 x 10^6 lymphocytes /ml of plasma. An initial panel of monoclonal antibodies was used to immune-phenotype T cells and their subgroups and B cells and their sub-groups. Immune-cytochemical detection of antigen was made using the ABC-AP, APAAP method. Activated B lymphocytes were defined as CD19 + cells, CD20, CD21, and CD23 and or CD138 surface markers. Activated T cells were identified with CD7, CD5, CD3, CD2, CD4, CD8.

The phenotype suggestive of B-CLL or monoclonal B cell lymphocytes was approximately equal numbers of CD5+ and CD19+ lymphocytes. Expected values to cytogenetic results will the deletion13q chromosome which can occur in more than 50% of patients and trisomy 12, which can occur in about 60 of patients.

Individual13q14 abnormalities have a relatively benign disease that usually manifests as stable or slowly progressive isolated lymphocytosis. Deletion in the short arm of chromosome 17 is associated with rapid progression, short remission, and decreased overall survival in chronic CLL. The 17p13 deletions are associated with loss of function of the tumor suppressor gene *p53* and deletions of bands 11q22-q23, associated with extensive lymph node, involvement aggressive disease and shorter survival. In the differential diagnosis of CLL we included Hairy cell leukemia, which is

moderately positive for surface membrane immunoglobulins of multiple heavy-chain classes and is typically negative for CD5 and CD21.

-CLL should also be distinguished from pro-lymphocytic leukemia, in which more than 65% of the cells are morphologically less mature pro-lymphocytes.

-Prolymphocytic leukemia has a typical phenotype that is positive for CD19, CD20, and surface membrane immunoglobulin but one-half will be negative for CD5. Large granular lymphocytic leukemia has a natural killer (NK) cell phenotype (CD2, CD16, CD56) or a T-cell immune type (CD2, CD3, CD8. The results are displayed in **[Table 1]**.

Normal concentration. ATP in T Cells	**Normal conc. ATP in B cells**	**Conc. ATP in T cells, malignant diseases**	**Conc. ATP B cells, malignant disease**	**Conc. ATP in B cells, CLL**	**Conc. ATP in T cells, CLL**
$\bar{x}$ = 1.39	**$\bar{x}$ =0.35**	**$\bar{x}$ == 3.06**	**$\bar{x}$ = 0.17**	**$\bar{x}$ =4.33**	**$\bar{x}$ = 0.09**
SD = 0.41	**SD = 0.42**	**SD = 0.46**	**SD = 0.45**	**SD =1.5**	**SD =1.7**

Table 1. *The concentrations of μM APT in malignant and chronic disease*

The mechanism involves inhibition of glycolytic ATP production via a Randle-like cycle while increased uncoupling renders cancers unable to produce compensatory ATP from respiration in the presence of intact tricarboxylic acid (TCA) enzyme. One mitochondrial adaptation to increased ROS is over-expression of the uncoupling protein 2 (UCP2) that has been reported in multiple human cancer cell lines Increased UCP2 expression was also associated with reduced ATP production in malignant oxyphilic mouse leukemia and human lymphoma cell lines.

Hypoxia reduces the ability of cells to maintain their energy levels because less ATP is obtained from glycolysis than from oxidative phosphorylation. Cells adapt to hypoxia by activating the expression of mutant genes in glycolysis. Severe hypoxia causes a high mutation rate, resulting in point mutations that may be explained by reduced DNA mismatch repairing activity.

The most direct induction of apoptosis caused by hypoxia is determined by the inhibition of the electron carrier chain from the inner membrane of the mitochondria. The lack of oxygen inhibits the transport of protons and thereby causes a decrease in membrane potential. Cell survival under conditions of mild hypoxia is mediated by a phosphoinositide-3 kinase (PIK3) using severe hypoxia or anoxia, and then cells initiate a cascade of events that lead to apoptosis.

After DNA damage, a very important regulator of apoptosis is the p53 protein. This tumor suppressor gene has mutations in over 60% of human tumors and acts as a suppressor of cell division. The growth-suppressive effects of p53 are considered to be mediated through the transcriptional trans-activation activity of the protein. In addition to the maturational state of the clonal tumor, the prognosis of patients with CLL is dependent on genetic changes within the neoplastic cell population.

The genetic changes can be identified by fluorescent probes to chromosomal using a technique referred to as fluorescent in situ hybridization (FISH). Chromosomal evaluation using FISH can identify certain chromosomal abnormalities of CLL that have prognostic significance.

The part of the short arm of chromosome 17 (del 17 q), with targets the cell cycle regulating protein p53, is particularly deleterious. This abnormality is found in 10% of patients with CCL and has a poor prognosis. Deletion of the long arm of chromosome 13(del 13q) is the most common genetic abnormality in CLL with roughly 50% of patients exhibiting this effect. These patients have the best prognosis and most will live many years without the need for therapy. Agents damaging DNA may increase the expression of p53 and its trans-activation activity, suggesting that p53 acts protect cells against the accumulation of mutants and their subsequent conversion to a malignant status.

Protein p53, in its normal form, acts in stopping the cell division and, if is damaged DNA, thus giving the cells the possibility of repairing DNA before the errors would duplicate and be passed on to the daughter cells. Antibodies to human p53 have been detected in patients with cancer. These antibodies are highly specific for malignant diseases and are rarely detected in healthy donors or patients having benign diseases.

This immune response is correlated with the presence of a p53 gene mutation, leading to the accumulation of an ineffective p53 protein in tumor cells with either tridimensional structure. Over-expression of normal p53

protein can result either in G1 arrest, mediated by p21 protein or in the induction of apoptosis. Hypoxia itself can also prevent apoptosis by inducing the expression of the anti-apoptotic protein IAP-2.

Blocked apoptosis from malignant diseases may be due to high ATP concentration originating from anaerobic metabolism. The difference of energy between anaerobic ATP in B lymphocytes from CLL and aerobic ATP in activated T lymphocytes from normal status and non-malignant diseases was 2.68 μM ATP, as an energetic transfer between T and B cells, initiates carcinogenesis by suppression anti-oncogene proteins, [7].

The measurement of ATP was made by standard principle of bioluminescence on automatic analyzer LKB, using ATP monitoring reagent, ATP Standard, (10^6 Mol ATP/ ml), buffer solution Tris-EDTA, TCA-EDTA lyse. All results were statistically analyzed by Excel program. T lymphocytes were obtained from the peripheral blood of healthy individual and from hospitalized patients with selected diseases from the departments of Internal Medicine and Oncology. Patient cohort was a total of 75 patients (50 males and 25 females) consisting of the following groups were examined: 25 patients (mean ages 55 ± 0.5)), with allergic diseases (allergic rhinitis, allergic dermatitis, chronic allergic asthma), 25 patients, (mean ages 58 ± 1.8) with non-hematopoietic malignant diseases (lung cancer, bone metastasis) and 25 patients with confirmed hematopoietic malignant disorders, in diagnosis of CLL.

In addition, 120 blood samples from apparently healthy donors (mean ages 40.02 ±12.01) were also examined. The May Grunwald-Giemsa method was used to determine the microscopic appearance of peripheral blood lymphocytes from patients with incipient CLL disease, who had not had any treatment or hematopoietic stem cell transplantation (HSCT). Morphologically, the cells resembled normal mature clonal B cells arrested in the B- cell differentiation pathway intermediate between pre-B cells and mature B cells lymphocytes although slightly larger, and more fragile when smeared onto a glass slide (smudge cells). Lymphocytes were separated from peripheral blood by centrifugation in a Ficoll gradient for 20 minutes at 2000 rcf/ minute.

Lysis of lymphocytes with TCA-EDTA was performed after cell counts were adjusted to 1 x 10^6 lymphocytes /ml of plasma. An initial panel of monoclonal antibodies was used to immune-phenotype T cells and their subgroups and B cells and their sub-groups. Immune-cytochemical detection of antigen was made using the ABC-AP, APAAP method.

Activated B lymphocytes were defined as CD19 + cells, CD20, CD21, and CD23 and or CD138 surface marker.

The phenotype suggestive of B-CLL or monoclonal B cell lymphocytes was approximately equal numbers of CD5+ and CD19+ lymphocytes. Expected values to cytogenetic results will the deletion13q chromosome that can occur in more than 50% of patients and trisomy 12, which can occur in about 60 of patients.

Individual13q14 abnormalities have a relatively benign disease that usually manifests as stable or slowly progressive isolated lymphocytosis. Deletion in the short arm of chromosome 17 is associated with rapid progression, short remission, and decreased overall survival in chronic CLL. The 17p13 deletions are associated with loss of function of the tumor suppressor gene *p53* and deletions of bands 11q22-q23, associated with extensive lymph node, involvement aggressive disease and shorter survival.

In the differential diagnosis of CLL we included:

-*Hairy cell leukemia*, which is moderately positive for surface membrane immunoglobulins of multiple heavy-chain classes and is typically negative for CD5 and CD21.

-CLL should also be distinguished from pro-lymphocytic leukemia, in which more than 65% of the cells are morphologically less mature pro-lymphocytes.

-Prolymphocytic leukemia has a typical phenotype that is positive for CD19, CD20, and surface membrane immunoglobulin but one half will be negative for CD5.

Mechanism involves inhibition of glycolytic ATP production via a Randle-like cycle while increased uncoupling renders cancers unable to produce compensatory ATP from respiration in the presence of intact tricarboxylic acid (TCA) enzyme. One mitochondrial adaptation to increased ROS is over-expression of the uncoupling protein 2 (UCP2) that has been reported in multiple human cancer cell lines Increased UCP2 expression was also associated with reduced ATP production in malignant oxyphilic mouse leukemia and human lymphoma cell lines Hypoxia reduces the ability of cells to maintain their energy levels, because less ATP is obtained from glycolysis than from oxidative phosphorylation. Cells adapt to hypoxia by activating the expression of mutant genes in glycolysis. Severe hypoxia causes a high mutation rate, resulting in point mutations that may be

explained by reduced DNA mismatch repairing activity.

The most direct induction of apoptosis caused by hypoxia is determined by the inhibition of the electron carrier chain from the inner membrane of the mitochondria. The lack of oxygen inhibits the transport of protons and thereby causes a decrease in membrane potential. Cell survival under conditions of mild hypoxia is mediated by phosphoinositide-3 kinase (PIK3) using severe hypoxia or anoxia, and then cells initiate a cascade of events that lead to apoptosis.

After DNA damage, a very important regulator of apoptosis is the p53 protein. This tumor suppressor gene has mutations in over 60% of human tumors and acts as a suppressor of cell division. The growth-suppressive effects of p53 are considered to be mediated through the transcriptional trans-activation activity of the protein. In addition to the maturational state of the clonal tumor, the prognosis of patients with CLL is dependent of genetic changes within the neoplastic cell population.

The genetic changes can be identified by fluorescent probes to chromosomal using a technique referred to as fluorescent in situ hybridization (FISH). Chromosomal evaluation using FISH can identify certain chromosomal abnormalities of CLL that have prognostic significance.

This abnormality is found in 10% of patients with CCL and has a pour prognosis. Deletion of long arm of chromosome 13(del 13q) is the most common genetic abnormality in CLL with roughly 50% of patients exhibiting this effect. These patients have the best prognosis and most will live many years without the need for therapy. Agents damaging DNA may increase the expression of p53 and its trans-activation activity, suggesting that p53 acts to protect cells against the accumulation of mutants and their subsequent conversion to a malignant status.

Protein p53, in its normal form, acts in stopping the cell division and, if is damaged DNA, thus gives to the cells the possibility of repairing DNA before the errors would duplicate and be passed on to the daughter cells. Antibodies to human p53 have been detected in patients with cancer. These antibodies are highly specific for malignant diseases and are rarely detected in healthy donors or patients having benign diseases.

This immune response is correlated with the presence of a p53 gene mutation, leading to the accumulation of an ineffective p53 protein in tumor cells with either tridimensional structure. Over-expression of normal p53 protein can result either in G1 arrest, mediated by p21 protein or in the

induction of apoptosis. Also, hypoxia itself ca also prevent apoptosis by inducing the expression of the anti-apoptotic protein IAP-2.

Blocked apoptosis from malignant diseases may be due to high ATP concentration originating from anaerobic metabolism. The difference of energy between anaerobic ATP in B lymphocytes from CLL and aerobic ATP.

CHAPTER VIII

ROLE OF VITAMINS IN THE GROWTH OF ENERGY CELLS

Vitamins are exogenous biological effectors indispensable for the growth, development and reproduction of all living things and humans, in catalytic quantities. I. The classical classification of vitamins is still used in medical practice. Water-soluble vitamins are thiamine, riboflavin, pyridoxine, niacin, pantothenic acid, folic acid, cobalamin, ascorbic acid, and p-amino-benzoic acid.

Thiamine (vitamin B1) exerts its action in the co-enzymatic form of thiamine pyrophosphate (TPP). TPP-dependent biochemical processes are represented by the reactions:

- **pyruvate --> acetyl CoA + CO2 ---→TPP alfa-ceto-glutarate dehydrogenase**
- **alfa-ceto-glutarate --> succinyl CoA + CO2 TPP trans-enolase**
- **xylulose-5-P + ribose-5-P ----> sedoheptulose-7-P + glyceride-aldehyde-3-P TPP**

The first two amino acids participate in the aerobic Krebs cycle and sedoheptulose-7-P participates in the pentose-phosphate pathway.

Riboflavin (vitamin B2) in the form of FMN and FAD (flavin-nucleotide and flavin-dinucleotide), respectively, has the role of a prosthetic group of flavin enzymes involved in numerous redox processes. Oxidases (aldehyde oxidase and xanthine oxidase) have FAD as coenzymes and dehydrogenases (acetyl CoA-DEH, succinate dehydrogenase and NADP2 dehydrogenase) have FAD-1 and FMN as coenzymes. Pyridoxine (vitamin B6) in active form is pyridoxal-5-phosphate which is formed by phosphorylation with ATP: **Pyridoxal-kinase pyridoxal + ATP ---> pyridoxal 5P + ADP**

Pyridoxal is involved in many amino acid metabolism reactions:

- decarboxylation of amino acids;
- amino acid transamination;
- elimination of H_2O from amino acids;
- elimination of H_2S from amino acids;
- degradation of amino acids. Niacin, (vitamin PP). The body can gain niacin by using the amino acid tryptophan as a precursor. Not only nicotinamide but also NAD results from this biosynthesis process.

NAD biosynthesis is dependent on pyridoxine and other B-complex vitamins, such as thiamine, riboflavin, and biotin. Niacin exerts its action after prior incorporation into the structure of NAD and NADP coenzymes. These coenzymes catalyze redox processes due to the property of nicotinamide embedded in the enzyme molecule to exist in both oxidized and reduced forms. highlights the intervention of ATP in the synthesis of NAD and NADP.

Pantothenic acid exerts its action after its previous incorporation into the acetylating coenzyme CoA. The structure of this coenzyme also includes cysteamine, phosphoric acid, ribose, and adenine as constituents. CoA is involved in all reactions involving any organic acid in tissues when ethyl-CoA-like structures of special metabolic importance are formed.

Biotin is the prosthetic group of enzymes involved in CO_2 fixation and trans-carboxylation reactions such as pyruvate carboxylase pyruvate + CO_2 ---> oxalacetate Folic acid, its structure includes pteroic acid, para-amino-benzoic acid and glutamic acid. In the form of tetra-hydrofoil acid, it acts as a coenzyme of transporter transferases. This fragment is involved in metabolic processes such as purine nucleotide biosynthesis, and reversible amino acid transformations. The main symptoms arising from the lack of amino acids are growth disorders and hematopoietic disorders, which lead to hypochromic anemia, leukopenia, and thrombopenia. A folic acid antagonist, methotrexate, is even used in the treatment of leukemias because it inhibits nucleic acid biosynthesis favored by folic acid.

Cobalamin (vitamin B12) consists of a pyrrole ring, a nucleotide, a phosphorus ribo-purine residue, a cobalt ion and cyanide (KN). It performs its biological role in the form of two coenzymes, 5-adenyl-cobalamin and methyl-cobalamin. Coenzyme formation involves the reduction of Co^{3+} to Co^{2+} and the uptake of d-adenosine from ATP or a methyl group from

adenosine methionine. It intervenes in erythropoiesis, respectively in the formation and maturation of erythrocytes, in the proper functioning of the nervous system and ensures the integrity of the mucous membranes of the oral cavity.

Ascorbic acid (vitamin C) is an acid, that contains 6 carbon atoms, two alcohol groups, and two enol groups. The main biochemical processes in which ascorbic acid is involved are:

a) microsomal redox reductions, as redox buffer against these processes;

b) the metabolism of steroid hormones that takes place in the endoplasmic reticulum;

c) the formation of polyunsaturated fatty acids that takes place at the level of the endoplasmic reticulum;

d) collagen formation hydroxylation with collagen formation. Fat-soluble vitamins are retinol, calciferol, tocopherols, and phylloquinone.

Retinol (vitamin A) is found in the form of provitamin in vegetables, green plants and animal products. The active forms of vitamin A are: retinol also called retinoic acid and vitamin A1. A compound called vitamin A2 is also found in fish liver. It intervenes in the process of vision, and the integrity of the epidermis and mucosa. Influences cell growth. Due to its ability to regulate cell growth, retinoic acid is used with good results in the treatment of neoplasms.

NAD + retinol ----> retinal ---> retinoic acid NADH + H$^+$

Calciferol (vitamin D) comes from animals and is formed in the body from cholesterol. Vitamin D has an anti-rickets action, a process dependent on the normal metabolism of calcium and phosphorus. In plasma, the product Ca2 + x H3PO42- should normally be greater than 48. In the intestine, the action of calciferol consists of a marked increase in calcium absorption based on the active transport of ATP.

It also participates in the synthesis of the bone matrix and the formation of the citrate ion, in the release of phosphorus and pyrophosphate from organic phosphates; due to the action of phosphatases, it stimulates the retro-resorption of phosphate and amino acids. All these processes proceed with high energy exchanges through the participation of ATP.

Toco-ferol (vitamin E) are spread in the plant, leaves, and cereal germs as well as in the animal body: liver, heart, and placenta. Due to their easily oxidizable structure, tocopherols can function as antioxidants, protecting against the oxidation of biologically active products. The strongest antioxidant activity is that of delta-tocopherol while the most intense anti-sterilizing action is alpha-tocopherol. Tocopherols intervene in the intermediate metabolism through the action they exert on the metabolism of nucleic acids and implicitly on the biosynthesis of proteins. It participates in the biosynthesis of heme, hemoproteins, and enzymes with hemin structure and thus in hematopoiesis. It influences the metabolism of fatty acids, especially polyunsaturated and cholesterol. Phyto-quinone (vitamin K).

Depending on the nature of the substances, several K vitamins can be distinguished. Some of them, namely vitamins K1 and K2, are found in nature in the vegetable form of green plants (spinach). Vitamin K is involved in the formation and release of II, VII, X, and XI. Due to their structural kinship with coenzyme Q, it also acts on the respiratory chain and oxidative phosphorylation through it. Other substances with vitamin action: Lipoic acid is a nutritional factor for certain organisms.

Its main function is its participation in the oxidative decarboxylation of keto acids under the action of the enzyme complex pyruvate dehydrogenase. Bioflavonoids (vitamin P). Among the most common flavonoids in nature is routine. Retinoid is a disaccharide consisting of rhamnose and glucose. Flavonoids are widespread in the plant kingdom, especially in flowers and fruits, accompanied by ascorbic acid in citrus fruits, rosehips, and blackcurrants. In humans, capillary permeability decreases as well as blood pressure in general. Ubiquinone (coenzyme Q) plays a role in cellular redox oxidation similar to that of pyridine or flavin coenzymes. It has a benzo-quinone structure and can exist in both oxidized and reduced forms.

Based on these reactions, ubiquinone can act as a carrier of hydrogen and electrons in the respiratory chain. Choline forms lectin and sphingomyelins, compounds that play an important role in lipid metabolism, fulfilling a structural role as well as a methyl group donor and acetylcholine precursor.

Vitamin F (essential fatty acids), is correct to be considered a complex of essential fatty acids in the sense that they are essential substances to the body and can not to synthesize and must be introduced into the body through food. However, they are needed in relatively large quantities, as they perform in addition to the function of biological effectors and the function of structural and energetic material.

The main essential fatty acids are linoleic acid and arachidonic acid. The administration of essential fatty acids lowers the level of cholesterol and determines the normal development of the metabolism of neutral fats. II. The intervention of vitamins and antioxidants in the prevention of carcinogenesis A nutritional deficiency and a vitamin deficiency characterizes most cancer patients. In the state phase, it has been observed that a vitamin deficiency can precede cancer. The presence of harmful substances in food or other environmental factors, their formation in the gastrointestinal tract or their appearance in the process of metabolic processing may be to some extent counteracted by a food intake rich in antioxidant protective factors.

Low levels of **vitamin A** have been shown to increase the risk of cancer. This relationship was independent of age and the number of cigarettes smoked (lung cancer). Recent studies have shown a high incidence of cancer in low-carotene patients. Carotene protects cell structures from oxidative reactions, thus limiting DNA damage.

Retinoids exert an antimutagenic action against the condensation of cigarette smoke, an anticancer action in the case of hydrocarbon administration (DMBA) and inhibition of retrovirus-induced tumours. Beta carotene also inhibits mutations in benzil-pyrene and mitomycin in the bone marrow. Most authors explain the mechanism of inhibition of chemical carcinogenesis by retinoids by blocking the action of the cancer phase in the cell population. Vitamin A is thought to have a beneficial effect only in the early stages of malignancy, in the advanced stages accelerating the process. Retinol has the property of inhibiting the oxidation of NADPH and ascorbate in microsomes and organelles in the liver, thus preventing the formation of lipo-peroxides in membranes.

Along with **vitamin E**, it has a stabilizing effect on membrane structures, which is essential for the proper functioning of the cell. At the same time, the metabolic activity decreases, decreasing the number of cells in the S cycle phase due to the blocking by the retinoids of the G1 phase in the cell mitotic cycle, preventing uncontrolled proliferation. It is estimated that people who eat large amounts of vegetables with yellow and green pigments have a lower incidence of cancer.

To explain the cytoprotective effect of retinoids in carcinogenesis, important functions are considered that they exert:

• blocks the activity of carcinogens;

• prevents the binding of carcinogens to cellular DNA;

• exerts a normalizing influence on the cellular phenotype potentiating a reversal of the processes;

• induces stabilization and increase of lysosomal and plasma permeability of normal and cancer cells;

• stimulates immunity.

Stopping at the last function it is believed that the immunological action of retinoids can be viewed in three ways:

1) retinoids do not have a direct influence on anticancer immunity but only change the surface of the cancer cell;

2) Retinoids primarily stimulate the activity of "killer" T lymphocytes against the cancer cell.

If the concentration of ATP in the cancer cell is very high to cope with the high rate of proton and DNA synthesis, in the cancer lymphocytes the concentration of ATP has raised too high parameters due to their intense activation by malignant cells. In animals that received vitamin A in the connective tissue around the cancerous area, the number of lymphocytes doubled compared to the control samples.

It is estimated that in the first stage of maturation, retinoids impede the process of chemical activation of the carcinogen. Furthermore, the binding of carcinogens to DNA becomes much more difficult in the presence of retinoids and as a result, the malignancy process is prevented. At this stage, retinoids manifest as normalizers of the cellular phenotype.

As is well known, the cancer cell is characterized by a lower pH than normal. Vitamin A ballooning lysosomes and releasing acid hydrolases will cause cancer cells to kill themselves. We emphasize that the modulation of the diet with the intake of vitamins cannot be a substitute for well-coded and effective treatments of surgery, radiotherapy, chemotherapy, and immunotherapy in cancer. In general, however, vitamins may also play a role in the complications of chemist-surgical treatments for cancer.

Vitamins B1, B2 and B6 are given in the neurological complications of cytostatic drugs. A protective effect against colon cancer has flavones and antioxidant factors (vitamins E, C, and Se).

The metabolic rate for colon cancer in the United States is higher in populations less exposed to sunlight. The risk of colorectal cancer was

inversely correlated with dietary vitamin D and calcium. The interest in the possible anticancer effect of antioxidants was determined by the fact that the formation of tumors is the result of the toxic action of oxy- or peroxy-radicals formed by oxidation of carcinogens, hydroxy-peroxide radicals, hydrogen peroxide and organic peroxides formed by by-products.

The obvious support for this hypothesis is that ionized radicals produce various organic peroxides in biological materials that have mutagenic and tumorigenic action and that diets with a high content of polyunsaturated fatty acids predispose to inducing carcinogenesis and that malonyl-aldehyde, a compound that breaks down peroxide acids. fat formed "in vivo" is carcinogenic.

Vitamin E1, a natural antioxidant of lipids, has been shown to reduce chemical carcinogenesis but to a lesser extent than most synthetic antioxidants. An example is the inhibition of the formation of peroxides of fatty acids by vitamin E, peroxides which are precursors of malonic aldehyde. In foods, especially those of plant origin, there is a wide range of phenolic compounds with antioxidant action.

Several authors have established a real antitumor action of some flavonoid derivatives on tumors of different etiologies as well as their ability to prevent metastases in some sarcomas. Recently, special importance has been given to selenium as a cytoprotective agent, as it has the effect of interrupting metabolic sequences that initiate neoplastic transformation due to the body's exposure to carcinogens. The carcinogenic action may be associated with its participation in the structure of glutathione peroxidase which protects cells from the degrading action of peroxides or corrects the alterations caused by chemical carcinogens. Selenium, sulfur amino acids and vitamin E have a synergistic action in protection against peroxides.

If in the deficiency of vitamin E the accumulation of H2O2 leads to the peroxidation of unsaturated lipids, the presence of selenium allows the direct transfer of electrons from glutathione to cytochromes. The step of producing hydrogen peroxide is thus avoided and as a result, cellular protection is ensured in this way. Tappel's research, in the year 1991 has shown that compounds with Se cause inhibition of peroxidation, decomposition of peroxides formed, removal of free radicals from chain reactions, and restoration of molecular integrity.

To a large extent, these effects are related to the activity of glutathione peroxidase, which depends on the exogenous ratio. It has been observed that

cytoplasmic absorption of Se means a low content of synthesized glutathione peroxidase (GSPH) proteins. There is a direct relationship between the cytoplasmic concentration between the two factors and the activity of normal cell differentiation. Se derivatives have been found to have applications in the treatment of cancer.

It should be noted that high doses of Se are toxic as they may inhibit mitosis t is in the embryo resulting in abnormal cartilage and bones, at concentrations greater than 0.25 ml by body weight. Natural sodium selenic following the cultivation of plants grown on land with selenium compounds is also possible. After atherosclerosis, cancer is the second morbid condition in which selenium protects antioxidants. Selenium also stimulates immunity, and moderates cell proliferation. It acts antimutagenic and anticancer. In animals, the protective effect was found even after the administration of carcinogens, in physiological doses selenium stops or delays the appearance of tumors caused by viruses from chemicals. Studies in Finland and the United States show a selenium deficiency several years before the onset of breast cancer.

This deficiency joins that of vitamins A, E and D whose preventive tumor effects have recently been highlighted. The decrease in selenium has also been reported as a predisposition to digestive tract cancers in which R J. Slamberger in the year 1987 discovers the lack of the protective enzyme, glutathione peroxidase, as in breast cancer in people who are low in polyunsaturated fats (vegetable fats).

In tissue cultures, selenium prevents the breakdown of DNA molecules by carcinogens by protecting chromosomes and genes. As a tumor agent, it intervenes in concentrations 30-60 times higher than in physiological ones. A biphasic level is found: at concentrations lower than 10-8 it stimulates cell proliferation and at concentrations lower than 10-5 M it inhibits it.

The prophylaxis of cancer and myocardial infarction by the ratio of this trace element is currently proposed. The reduced intake of some people is due to the current preferences for meat, sweets and fats with fewer vegetables and black bread. The current preparation "Selenase" can be administered in doses of 200 mg/day orally and by injection. Selenatropic exaggeration, however, should be tempered given the range of toxic and therapeutic doses. Ensuring a normal concentration in the body through proper nutrition, according to the activity performed as well as according to the season is, as people say, "clean health". Increased alcohol consumption, smoking and vitamin C deficiency in the body are risk factors for

oesophagal cancer.

A diet rich in vitamin C blocks the conversion of nitrates and nitrogen-containing compounds to potential risk factors for cancer. This inhibition is very important in the prevention of gastric cancer, with vitamin C being recommended in chemotherapy in doses of 200 mg/day. In addition to the known antioxidant action, ascorbic acid intervenes in hydroxide reactions, participating in the detoxification of xenobiotics, including carcinogens by promoting their metabolism.

Vitamin C occurs both in the first phase of oxidant metabolism and in the second phase, with an important role being given to gluconic acid and sulfur as conjugating agents. Vitamin F is the group of unsaturated fatty acids that play the role of co-ferments and which together with vitamins B6, and E (as vitamins) is necessary for the synthesis of fats. Some research gives an important place to unsaturated fatty acids in the prevention of cancer. Vitamin F is involved in the metabolism of cholesterol and the metabolism of certain fatty acids. In its absence, liver function and the antitoxic power of the liver are disturbed. Vitamin F also helps maintain the normal permeability of cell membranes, especially the intestines.

Thus, according to researcher C. Kosmine, under the influence of vitamin F deficiencies, the intestinal wall becomes abnormally permeable, allowing microorganisms with weak pathogenic power but armed with toxins to pass daily. In a predisposed part of the body, thanks to an additional permeabilizing factor, the hormone in case of breast cancer, a carcinogen in case of the smoker, etc., a tumor is formed.

Therefore, suppression of avitaminosis F leads to the inhibition of intestinal microbial migration. The body's need to build an antimicrobial defence tissue involved in antitumor defence would result from an F and B6 deficiency. An internal medical treatment tending to suppress these deficiencies, therefore, appears necessary as a complement to the classical methods and as a progression in antitumor therapy.

At the end of this chapter we summarize the main mechanisms involved in the prevention of malignancy:

- increasing the body's antitumor resistance capacity by correct vitamins;
- regulation of food poisoning processes;
- promoting an aerobic cellular regime through a systematized physical

regime in a natural environment, negatively aerated;

• competitive inhibition of carcinogens in the body.

Research by Wattenberg and others has shown that inhibition of cancer is f possible, in some cases experimentally proving that inhibition of the promotion stage may occur. As Voiculeţ and D. Niculescu have shown, substances that inhibit this stage can suppress the expression of the transformed cell phenotype. Moreover, it has been established that among the promotion inhibitors there are substances capable of inducing even the terminal differentiation of some malignant cells, respectively to cause the reversal of the malignant phenomenon to the tumor one. These biologically active substances include:

1) prostaglandin synthetase inhibitors: carotenes, retinoids;

2) antioxidant (Se, vit. C, El, vegetable phenols);

3) isothiocyanates and titanates in general;

4) coumarins and lactones;

5) oxidase-inducing substances and inhibitors with mixed microsomal functions;

6) a normal physiological intake of amino acids: histidine, asparagine, glutamic acid, valine and arginine, which reduce DNA mutations, **[Figure 3]**, [8].

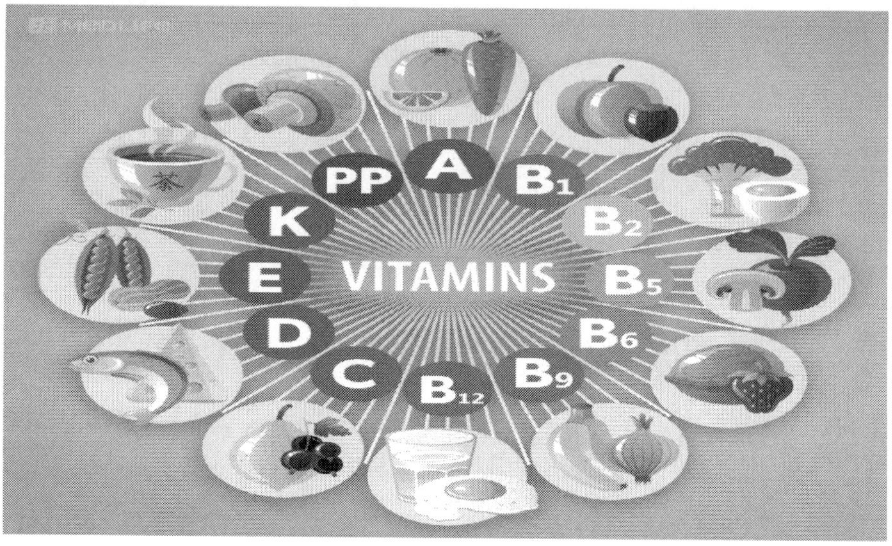

Figure 3. *Vitamins: a nutritional organic molecule, (Plantlet)*

CHAPTER IX

SIGNIFICANCE OF THE ATP-MG COMPLEX IN ENDOCRINE REGULATION

Hormones are endogenous biochemical effects secreted directly into the blood by specialized cells of the endocrine glands in the endocrine system or endocrine cells in the individualized anatomical structure. Transported by blood to the organs of the target effects, they exert a stimulating, integrating action on physiological and metabolic or inhibitory processes. In target cells, needle hormones are based on two main mechanisms:

1. Activation or inhibition of enzymes by cyclic AMP or cyclic GMP;

2. Genetically controlled enzymatic induction or repression. Many hormones, especially with a non-steroidal structure, such as adrenaline, glucagon and other polypeptide hormones exert their action very quickly (30-60 ") by fixing them on specific receptors on the target cell membrane and thus activate the enzyme adenyl cyclase or Adenyl-cyclase catalyzes the conversion of ATP to cyclic AMP cAMP can activate, through proteins, enzyme-dependent ATP systems, can influence cell membrane permeability and as such cellular transformations. an enzyme called phosphodiesterase.

Adenyl-cyclase phosphodiesterase ATP --> AMP-c -----> AMP
Mg adenyl-cyclase hormone --> Membrane receptor --> ATP -> cAMP + p
protein kinase hormone --> membrane receptor ----> ATP ----> ADP + p-protein

Among the complete non-steroidal hormones, insulin is of particular importance in intermediate metabolism. Insulin exerts a metabolic action based on its ability to function as a cyclic anti-AMP factor. In organs sensitive to the action of insulin, it increases the permeability of the cell wall for monosaccharides, amino acids, and fatty acids, thus increasing their cytoplasmic concentration and the possibility of metabolism (adipose tissue, liver, and muscle). Insulin induces the biosynthesis of key glycolysis enzymes: hexokinase, phosphofructokinase, and phospho-enol-pyruvate-

kinase.

This activates both glycolysis and the Krebs cycle. Under the influence of insulin, the degradation of glucose by pentose-phosphates is also increased, through which important amounts of NADPH2 are formed. Insulin stimulates the biosynthesis of found acids as well as fats in general.

The effect of insulin on protein metabolism is to stimulate protein biosynthesis due to increased penetration of amino acids into cells as well as increased RNA synthesis in cells with specific receptors. Through its mitochondrial action, insulin intervenes directly in the ATP-AMP relationship and conditions the coupling of tissue respiration with oxidative phosphorylation. Highlighting its action on mitochondrial contraction, through experimental work, altering its cycle in diabetes, highlights the integration of the above assumptions in the molecular theory of insulin.

It has been found that in experimental diabetes there is an alteration of the swelling-contraction cycle of mitochondria. The described effect is found in hepatic muscle mitochondria in normal cells, where ATP-induced mitochondrial contraction in the presence of insulin is greater than ATP-induced contraction in the presence of cysteine, **[Figure 3]**.

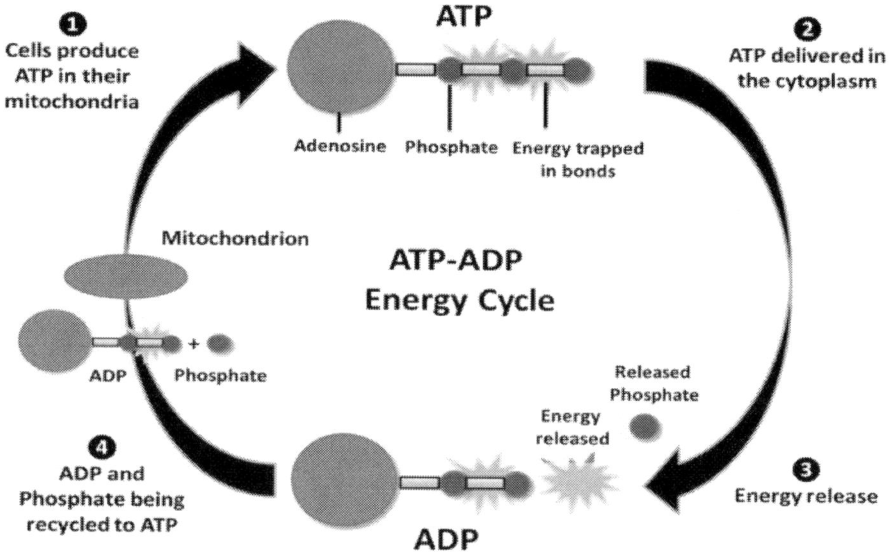

Figure 3. *Health and ergogenic potential of adenosine-5'-triphosphate in the delivery of cells energy*

Glucagon is the hormone antagonist of insulin and acts on the target organs, especially the liver and adipose tissue via the cAMP-adenylate-cyclase system. Parathyroid hormone, parathyroid hormone, mobilizes Ca2 + and P2 + from the bones, induces osteoblast inhibition and stimulates osteoclast activity.

Ca and P mobility in the bone can be explained by the influence that the parathyroid hormone exerts on glycolysis and the Krebs cycle in osteoclasts. These phenomena lead to the accumulation of citric acid and other organic acids that chelate Ca from the bones, thus favoring its mobilization. Parathyroid hormone is involved in mitochondrial cellular respiration and active transport of Ca in the mitochondria. Calcitonin inhibits osteoclast activation and stimulates osteoblasts activation and thus Ca and P deposits in the bone system. Stimulation of bone mineralization causes a decrease in the blood concentration of Ca and P. Thymus hormones (thymic, thymine, thymopectin I and II) stimulate the proliferation of lymphoid cells and the differentiation of T lymphocytes, thus intervening in the body's immune processes.

Hormone Erythropoietin accelerates the formation and maturation of erythrocytes, especially in hypoxic conditions. Prostaglandins are derived from fatty acids with 20 carbon atoms that may have 3.4 or 5 C = C double bonds in the molecule. The most common precursor of prostaglandins is the widely used arachidonic acid in tissues. Under the influence of cyclooxygenase, it is converted to a cyclic endoperoxide (PGG2), the immediate precursor of prostaglandins, thromboxane and prostacyclin. Prostaglandins act on both adrenal-ciklase and guanyl cyclase, influencing the synthesis of cAMP and cGMP. Through these secondary messengers, prostaglandins influence the secretion of endocrine glands such as the thyroid, adrenal glands, and parathyroid glands. Excitation or damage to cell membranes also triggers prostaglandin biosynthesis by releasing unsaturated fatty acids from phospholipids, which results in active stimulation of neighbor cells in the same tissue or tissues. Other hormones such as bradykinin, acetylcholine, and histamine, also stimulate prostaglandin synthesis.

Prostaglandins are involved in inflammatory processes and some non-steroidal anti-inflammatory drugs (aspirin, indomethacin) justify, at least in part, their pharmacodynamic action on their ability to inhibit prostaglandin biosynthesis. Thyroid hormones are derived from the amino acids thyroxine (thyroxine, T4), and tri-iodo-thyroxine (T3). Thyroid hormones exert multiple effects on the body to ensure the regulation, integration and coordination of the main physiological functions of the body, **[Figure 4].**

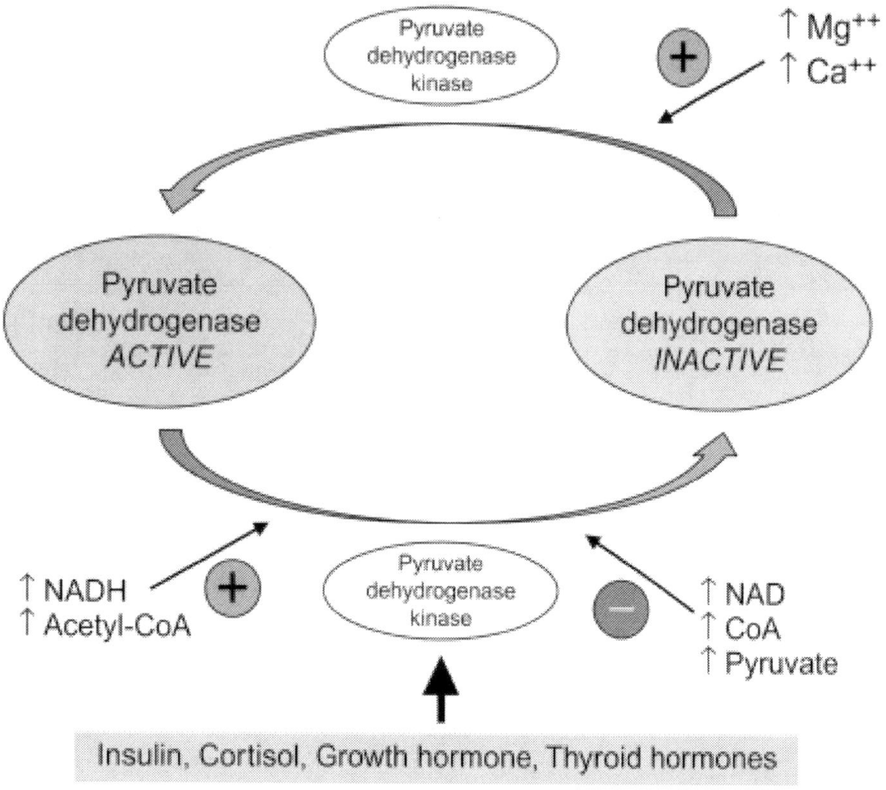

Figure 4. *Adenosine Diphosphate Magnesium in energetic mitochondrial activity*

Their somatotropic action is due to the role of thyroid hormones in the biosynthesis and distribution of structural and enzymatic proteins as well as nucleic acids. It creates a hypercatabolic state. At even higher concentrations, thyroid hormones cause the decoupling of oxidative phosphorylation with a decrease in respiratory rate (P / O). Mitochondrial oxidation reductions are also activated because thyroid hormones cause changes in the permeability of mitochondrial membranes leading to mitochondrial ballooning.

Low hormone levels also lead to a decoupling of phosphorylation with disruption of aerobic metabolism. Therefore, cancer may be due to hypofunction or glandular hyperfunction that creates intracellular metabolic conditions for the expression of chromosomal oncogenes. Through the hormones mentioned and with a large number of enzyme systems, which

they influence, the thyroid hormones control the entire intermediate metabolism.

Catecholamine biosynthesis takes place in the mitochondria of chromaffin cells in the adrenal medulla and the mitochondria of peripheral and central neurons when L-tyrosine is transformed into dopamine. Then, the synthesis continues extra-mitochondrially when dopamine changes to noradrenaline which is metabolized to adrenaline. The physiological role of catecholamines is based on their stimulatory action on adrenergic receptors. The metabolic action of adrenaline is exerted through receptors that are associated with adenyl cyclase on the target cell membrane.

By stimulating the cAMP system, adenyl cyclase influences carbohydrate metabolism by intensifying it in the opposite direction to the action of insulin, adrenaline being the most active natural antagonist of insulin. Thus, adrenaline has a global hyperglycemic effect because it accentuates phosphorylation, activating phosphorylase-b-kinase. This enzyme catalyzes the conversion of phosphorylase "b" to more active phosphorylase "a".
phosphorylase b 2 phosphorylase b + 4 ATP -----phosphorylase a + 4 ADP
kinases

Under the action of phosphorylase "a" glycogen cleaves to form glucose-1-P, which in the liver and muscles oxidizes intensely to CO_2 and H_2O, leading to a calorific effect. Noradrenaline does not influence phosphorylase "b". Both catecholamines cause an increase in lipolysis in adipose tissue via cAMP. Due to their glycogenolytic, lipolytic, and calorigenic effects, the global activation of catecholamines is catabolizing.

The main biochemical mechanism by which catecholamines act, in their capacity as b adrenergic receptor activators, is to increase the biosynthesis of cAMP, a process in which ATP, GTP and possibly other organ or tissue-dependent factors also participate. Steroid hormones. Structurally, it is derived from the so-called C_7H_{28} hydrocarbon also known as steran (cyclo-pentane-perhydro-phenanthrene).

Hormones secreted by the endocrine glands are taken up by plasma receptors that carry them to target organs and cells. nuclear receptors and intervene especially in the transcription of the genetic message. This stimulates the synthesis of proteins and especially of specific enzymes whose formation forms the basis of the physiological action of steroid hormones.

After steroid hormones exert their biological action in their cells, their catabolism takes place for excretion, with the participation of the redox chain leading to the appearance of hydroxylated compounds. Estrogen hormones (estrone, estriol, estradiol) control the synthesis of structural and functional proteins in the transcription of the genetic message in the uterine mucosa. Progestin hormones influence the structure of the vaginal mucosa, the development of mammary glands and glandular acini by the same molecular mechanism. Increased progesterone levels in the blood cause a decrease in either direct or long hypothalamus,

FSH and LH secretion through a short or long feedback process. Testosterone, the male sex hormone itself, secreted by the testicle and in small amounts by the adrenal cortex and ovary, is transported to the target organs by blood bound to a specific transport protein. In target cells, under the action of a 5th testosterone reductase enzyme, testosterone is reduced to the 5th α dihydroxy-testosterone, the active form.

The main mechanism by which it plays its complex physiological role is to regulate and control the synthesis of structural and functional proteins in the transcription of the genetic message from DNA to RNA. Testosterone can also influence the permeability of cell membranes as well as the activity of some enzymes through allosteric mechanisms. The anabolic effect of sex hormones is explained by their influence on protein metabolism with increasing muscle mass with muscle hypertrophy.

We emphasize the participation of testosterone in the lymphocyte system in the sense of physiological stimulation of helper T cells. Adrenal cortical hormones have glucocorticoid function, mineralocorticoid function and sex hormone function. Like all steroid hormones, corticosteroid hormones exert their action inside the target organs, influencing the biosynthesis of DNA-dependent proteins.

The hypothalamic-pituitary-adrenal cortex axis is the main mechanism that ensures the adaptation of homeostasis, the balance of the body concerning all environmental factors. Corticosteroids intervene in the adaptation to environmental hazards and overloads. Cortisol and hormones with glucocorticoid action strongly influence carbohydrate metabolism and stimulate glycogenesis by inhaling phosphorylation and activating glycogen synthesis.

It influences gluconeogenesis by activating some enzymes with an important role in gluconeogenesis, such as pyruvate carboxylase, phosphoenolpyruvate

carboxylase, fructose 1-6 bi-phosphatase, glucose-6-phosphatase. It also exerts a hyperglycemic action on protein metabolism, with cortisol acting differently, stimulating the biosynthesis of enzymatic proteins and the liver and inhibiting them in peripheral organs and tissues. In lipid metabolism, glucocorticoids intervene by exerting a global lipolytic action. Aldosterone influences mineral metabolism, the exchange of Na-K, producing activation of the sodium pump.

The complex biological and especially anti-inflammatory and immunosuppressive action of glucocorticoids, as cell membrane stabilizers and especially stimulators of suppressor T cells, increases in parallel with the induced cAMP concentration, due to the action of ACTH on the adrenal cortex. Based on some mechanisms, corticosteroids influence carbohydrate, lipid, protein, and mineral metabolism, regulating the activity of apparatus and systems. Steroidogenesis has been shown to increase in parallel with the intracellular concentration of cAMP. It is accepted that the stage influenced by cAMP in the adrenal gland is that of converting cholesterol to pregnenolone.

There is evidence that some actions of prostaglandins, calcium, and insulin, are also manifested through cAMP, the hormones mentioned also acting on adenyl cyclase or phospho-di-esterase (usually by replacing it). The highest and most complex level of regulation and control of physiological and metabolic processes in the body is the central nervous system and the vegetative system. Across the entire nervous system, acetyl-coline plays the role of a typical neurotransmitter.

Acetylcholine, in the nerve cell, is synthesized from choline and acetyl CoA under the action of cholinesterase with the participation of ATP: **ATP-aze-Choline + Acetyl CoA ----. >Acetylcholine ATP -----> AMP + P-P**

Nerve tissue is endowed with enzymatic equipment necessary for the metabolic processes that take place at this level: carbohydrate and lipid metabolism. It also contains respiratory chain enzymes. Maintaining nerve activity requires a permanent supply of energy, provided by ATPase, an enzyme that breaks down one of the macro-energetic bonds in ATP. Through the action of ATPase, energy is also released in the synthesis processes of acetylcholine and glutamine.

Without claiming to deplete the full range of neurosecretory, glandular or tissue hormones, in this chapter I wanted to highlight the implications of certain hormones in cell catabolism or anabolism. In conclusion, I

emphasize that hormonal regulation takes place in hierarchically organized themes, and at the highest level is the nervous system which through endorphins and hypothalamic bodies controls the activity of the pituitary gland in terms of somatotropic, endocrine-tropic and antidiuretic.

Also, the endocrine gland, the epiphysis, through the endocrine cells regulates the activity of the endocrine glands and influences the functions of the effector organs, by directly or indirectly, positively or negatively, controlling the enzymatic reactions that take place inside the cells of the tissue and organs. On the other hand, through a self-regulating mechanism of feedback (feedback), the concentration of products resulting in a metabolic stage can positively or negatively influence the development of processes at higher regulatory levels, [9].

CHAPTER X

BIOENERGETIC INTERFERENCE BETWEEN NORMAL AND MALIGNANT

Given that the predominant anaerobic metabolism is restored in the malignant cell, we will comparatively analyze the development of anaerobic glycolysis, both in the cancer cell and in the normal cell. In the normal cell, modelled on the liver cell, glucose metabolism always begins with phosphorylation of glucose G-6-P, the reaction being catalyzed by hexokinase (km) and glucokinase (KM) with the participation of ATP which will be converted to ADP.

G-ATP-....... ADP + G-6-P
Hexokinase or Glucokinase enzyme

The reaction is directly irreversible but becomes reversible with another enzyme, glucose-6-phosphatase. G-6-P G-6-P-cabbage G In the normal cell, hexokinase or glucokinase is inhibited by the high concentration of glucose, free fatty acids and glucose-6-phosphatase, an enzyme which in turn is inhibited by the high concentration of inorganic phosphate. In the malignant cell, G-6-P phosphorylation is performed only by hexokinase with the participation of ATP and the enzymes glucokinase and gluco-6-phosphatase are inhibited.

The reaction is strictly irreversible, once the glucose starts on this path it does not return. PHI H. G-6-P junction F-6-P catalyzed by phospho- hexo-isomerase is reversible in both normal and malignant cells. The conversion of F-6-P to F-1-6-P under the action of phosphofructokinase is again irreversible in both cell types directly. In the normal cell, phosphofructokinase is inhibited by high concentrations of ATP, AGL and citrate, and high concentrations of AMP and ADP stimulate the reaction.

None of these factors inhibits phosphofructokinase in the cancer cell. In the normal cell, the reversibility of the F-1-6-P;> F-6-P reaction provided by phosphofructo-1-6 diphosphatase does not occur if ATP is present in excess cytoplasm. The transformation of F-1-6-P.> PEP comprises a complex of

reactions in both cells catalyzed by aldolase, glycerol-aldehyde dehydrogenase, and phosphoglucomutase.

The PEP- PK pyruvate reaction is directly irreversible in the normal cell and strictly irreversible in the malignant cell where pyruvate carboxylase is inhibited. In the normal cell pyruvate kinase (PK), an enzyme that converts phosphoenolpyruvate to pyruvic acid is inhibited by high concentrations of pyruvic acid, citrate, ATP, NAD and the intensification of the Krebs cycle at the rate of oxidation.

The final glycolysis reaction of converting pyruvate to lactate is reversible in both normal and malignant cells and catalyzed by the same enzyme, LDH. However, it has been observed that LDH isoenzymes predominate in neoplastic processes. The energy-consuming and therefore uneconomical process in the normal cell (glycolysis) is now becoming economical in the cancer cell. In the normal cell for a certain value of ATP concentration, a balance is established between glycolysis (catabolism) and gluconeogenesis (anabolism).

The energy load of the cell, if it is between 1-2.5, directs the metabolism of glucose through catabolism or anabolism depending on the energy requirements of the cell in the aerobic environment. In the cancer cell, this balance is raised to a higher parameter and the high value of ATP no longer becomes inhibitory as does the low concentration of cAMP. Regarding aerobic catabolism, the Krebs cycle is fed with compounds from metabolism, very different and even some constituents of the cycle serve to synthesize important cellular components:

• oxalic acid is a precursor of gluconeogenesis;

• alpha-ceto-glutaric acid can lead to the formation of glutamine and in this form participates in the biosynthesis of purine bases;

• succinic acid, fumaric acid and malic acid are also precursors of gluconeogenesis;

• succinyl CoA is the precursor of heme in hemoglobin and cytochrome C.

In traditional folk medicine, cases have been cited when cancer patients were cured after 2 months by consuming 100 gr daily. of raw cabbage juice. This vegetable is rich in Ca oxalate. By dissolving calcium oxalate and oxalic acid in vivo, amino support is created for the Krebs cycle, the predominant onset of which would cause malignant reversion to normal,

without destroying the cancer cell.

The cancer cell secures its synthesis factors predominantly from glycolysis and the pentose-phosphate pathway. What remains characteristic of the cancer cell is the change in aerobic to anaerobic metabolism. This change could be dictated by the expression of oncogenes stimulated by toxic factors or initially, the toxic factors could lead to the onset of anaerobiosis, and cellular oncogenes would be expressed against this background.

Glycolysis in normal cells:

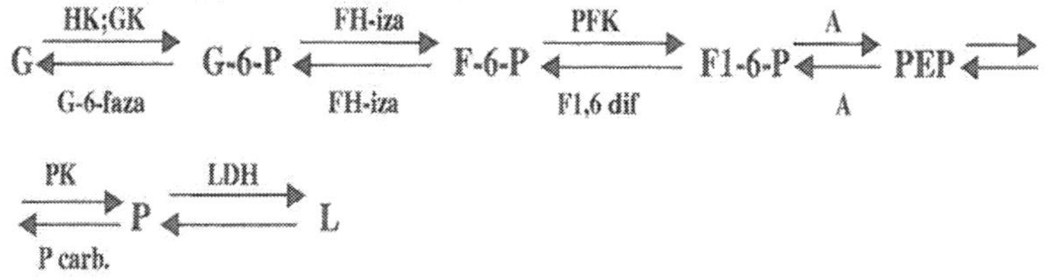

Glycolysis in malignant cells:

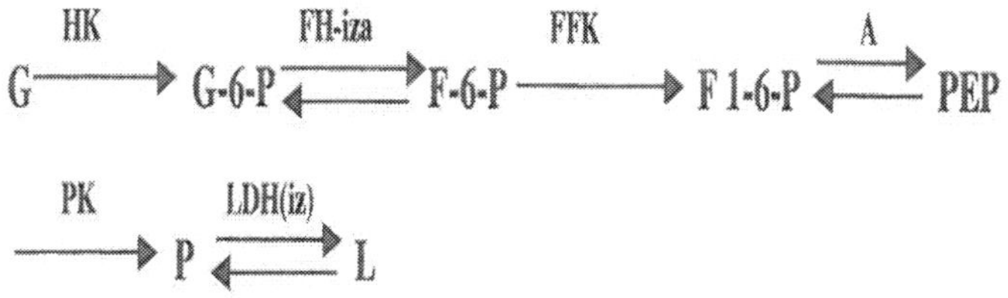

Last option, namely that initially the cellular infrastructures, would be damaged by toxic factors, infectious or permanent, even in small but cumulative doses. As oncogenes are older due to phylogeny, they may be the last to withstand aggression. The discovery of Peyton Rous at the turn of the century, the virus that causes bird sarcoma, was the first confirmation of the viral hypothesis behind cancer. Protein phosphorylation is known to be a normal process in cell metabolism. The synthesis of phosphorylated proteins with enzymatic characters is determined by a group of genes called normal proto-oncogenic cells.

Several 40 such genes have been isolated, stating that they are involved in the development of the cell cycle by regulating the multiplication and differentiation or maturation of cells. Since basic sequences similar to those

in proto-oncogenes have been found in simple life forms, they are considered to be very old and therefore essential for life.

Their transformation into oncogenes is possible in two ways:

1) By structural mutation when the products it encodes become normal;

2) By exaggerated multiplication or excessive activity with elaboration in large quantities of products that intervene in the cellular metabolism.

Recent genetic research has revealed genes with an inhibitory role: antioncogenes. Because their exact location is unknown, these progenitor antagonists have been called suppressor genes. There are genes that, if inactivated or disrupted, are prone to cancer. There is a double system in which excessive activation of stimulant genes is as harmful as the inactivation of inhibitory genes,

After the 1970s, the possibility of cancer was highlighted by altering the genetic structures, respectively the DNA in the nucleus. It is necessary to combine two factors: genetic predisposition and exogenous toxins. These toxins can be mutagenic clinical substances, ionizing radiation, viruses, etc. Simply put, malignant tissue appears as a disorder of cell proliferation and maturation that results in completely normal shapes, structures, and functions.

Structurally distorted, malignant cells escape the control of the body, and become autonomous, multiplying infinitely without ever maturing until death. In the form of proto-oncogenes, they control proliferation and differentiation (maturation) but by the transformation they become carcinogenic.

Several explanations have been found in this regard:

• localized mutations;

• changing a base in the structure of DNA with the introduction of other amino acids in the products produced.

Consequent, these products of the respective genes are either functionally blocked or partially modified;

• amplifying the number of copies of a gene. This mechanism has been found in colon cancer;

• the movement of a proto-oncogene in the vicinity of an intensely active gene; for example, immunoglobulin genes in lymphoid cells;

• translocation, dislocation, rupture of a portion of two non-homologous chromosomes followed by reciprocal exchange of segments;

• introduction of an abnormal portion into a proto-oncogene. Suppressor genes slow down the transcription of their progenitors and exert an opposite effect on the target molecules at which the transcription of genetic information into a messenger ribonucleic acid for specific protein synthesis occurs.

It was known beforehand that the replacement of a defective chromosome stops the malignancy of the cell. This suggests that the malignant cell has one or more defective genes that are essential for a normal life. The loss of inhibitory genetic information is as harmful as the over-function of oncogenes that stimulate cell proliferation.

The presence of suppressor genes has been accurately detected at the chromosomal level. For cancer to occur, both the suppressor gene inherited from the father and the mother must be altered. In the case of a single gene failure, there is only one predisposition. Here are some chromosomal deficiencies found in some human tumours: • lung cancer, Cr 3 p (p = short arm)

• rectal cancer, Cr 3 p

• breast cancer, Cr 11 p

• colon cancer, Cr 17 p

• LGC cancer, LA = Cr 9 q (q = long arm)

• retinoblastoma cancer, Cr 13 q

• gastric cancer, Cr 13 q

• neuroblastoma cancer, Cr 1 p

• meningioma cancer, Cr 22 q

In other words, where the individual inherits both defective suppressor genes, from mother and father, endogenous cancer is established, and if the inherited genetic defect is restricted to only one suppressor gene,

carcinogenesis is established under the influence of toxic, infectious, chemical, and physical factors **[Figure 5]**.

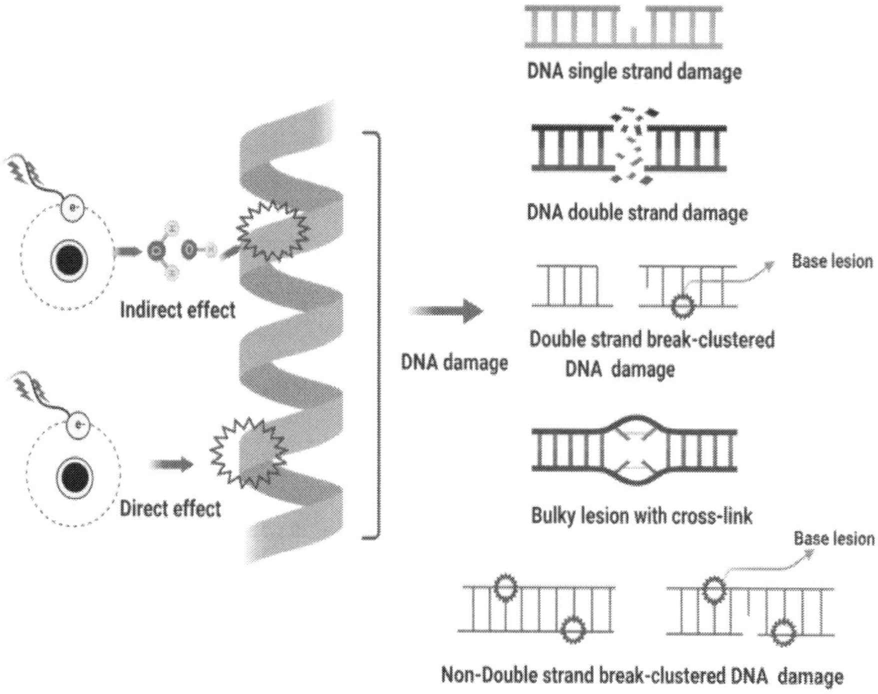

Figure 5. F*actors, especially certain environmental hazards such as toxic heavy metals and ionizing radiation, have been intensively studied and found to cause serious DNA damage*

The suppressor genes can also be altered by viruses, which has been shown not only in viruses well known as malignant in vitro, such as adenoviruses but also in some benign ones belonging to the herpes group (involvement of Epstein-Barr virus in nasopharyngeal cancer).

Whyte et al, 1995, discovered in the adenovirus the E1A gene responsible for malignant cells in mammals. These viruses malign not only by modifying the suppressor gene but also by blocking its product, which is equivalent to altering the genes. For example, the carcinogenic adenovirus synthesizes a complex of three cellular proteins, of which E1A is a protein identical to the product developed by the Rb genes. The Rb gene encodes a phosphoprotein that locates in the nucleus to bind to DNA. This

phosphoprotein limits cell proliferation in both the retina and other tissues. Alteration of the Rb gene is a key factor in the onset of retinoblastoma.

Wilms tumor (embryonic carcinoma of the kidney) is caused by alteration of the 11 q 13 genes and the introduction of the normal chromosome 11 into the cells prevents the appearance of the neoplasm. In meningioma, the lack of a suppressor gene was found on the long arm of chromosome 22, the benignity being explained by the loss of a single copy of the gene. This situation was found in acoustic neurinoma in which a suppressor gene suffers.

Given these aspects, we can conclude that proto-oncogenes become oncogenic through structural changes and non-physiological activations under conditions of inadequate anaerobic metabolism. Inhibitory suppressor genes whose absence or inactivation due to their damage or non-expression in the metabolic conditions created by chronic cellular suffering at some point generate this disorder.

Substitution of normal proteins normally produced by suppressor genes or the creation of metabolic conditions for the physiological repair of damaged genes would be physiological antitumor procedures without side effects that would oppose uncontrolled tumor proliferation.

It is believed that in the process of carcinogenesis, the mitochondria of normal cells would be attacked by carcinogens and partially damaged, and the DNA would be better protected by the double nuclear membrane. Suppressor gene damage would occur later than mitochondrial damage. Subsequently, the nuclear barriers will give way and the DNA will be functionally damaged (carcinogenesis) or physically damaged (cancer installed) by reactivating oncogenes that find their natural environment of expression in a phylogenetic-scale anaerobic environment similar to the primary one.

If the cell were permanently restored to its original state of aerobiosis by the cessation of toxic factors, the cell could find the potential to repair its DNA through its enzymes, especially DNA ligase with the participation of ATP.

The importance of DNA in the development of vital processes both as a structural element, chromosomal and functional component, preservation and transmission of genetic information, and protein biosynthesis justifies the consideration of this component as the ultimate main target of toxic, physical, chemical, biological factors in general and radiation ionic in particular. Viral factors induce mutations or express cellular oncogene by

insertion into cell DNA with gene dislocation or nuclear hybridization. The structural changes that radiation produces in DNA in the cellular context may explain the obvious macroscopic effects, biochemical and genetic functional disturbances, and even cell death.

The energy required to induce a single single-chain rupture in mammals is 50 eV-100 eV if it was done in an oxygen atmosphere. The irradiated cell can recover by removing sublethal lesions. Experiments have shown that the potentially lethal lesion in the cell can be altered or converted by changing environmental conditions immediately after irradiation.

This phenomenon has been called cell restoration or restoration. The repair mechanisms consist of completing the rupture ("gap") caused by an enzymatic excision and each of them contains several stages of reaction: the separatory replication, the phenomenon of "defect of replicative synthesis" of DNA and the reunion of the strands that will eventually lead to the restoration of the contents of the broken polynucleotide chain. These processes are catalyzed by pre-existing enzymes in the cells, enzymes that promptly intervene in the recognition and repair of the lesion. Of these, the DNA ligase that acts for the act is deliberately detached.

It is known that 228 kcal and redox potential of about 10 eV arise from the Krebs cycle coupled with oxidative phosphorylation. If 50-100 eV from radiation is added to this potential, it means that the sum of the accumulated energy becomes harmful to the mitochondria and the cell nucleus. This harmful overload could also explain the cellular metabolic overload with destructive effects due to the very high rate of catabolism of superstructures in the body's stresses.

High aerobic metabolism at high parameters eventually leads to the installation of anaerobic metabolism. The aerobic change in anaerobic metabolism was observed by the Japanese in altitude adaptation experiments. Exposure to hypobaric hypoxia corresponding to an altitude above 6000 m initially causes, before the adaptation of the organism, a decrease of the ATP reserve and an increase of cAMP that will activate more intensely phosphofructokinase.

A marked increase in lactate and uric acid in exposure above 6000 m indicates that glycolysis is essential and that the aerobic metabolism of fatty acids is not essential for the generation of ATP in tissues in the acute phase of exposure of the non-acclimatized organism. Exposure to a high hypoxic altitude causes a metabolic and biochemical change and causes a change in

the concentration of O2 in the blood and tissues. Once the adaptation is made, there is a stimulation of the oxidative metabolism given by the intensification of the use of O2 in the mitochondria from the cellular oxygen reserves. Then there is the change in the ATP-forming reaction of anaerobic glycolysis to oxidative metabolism.

These results suggest that metabolic acclimatization to hypobaric hypoxia by repeated exposure at progressive altitudes up to 6000 m induces a change in energy metabolism from anaerobic glycolysis in the pre-adaptation period to aerobic metabolism when adaptation has been made. Returning to a normal altitude, this increased functional capacity of all cells in the body is maintained for a maximum of 21-28 days, after which the cellular parameters return to the previous normal forms. Can we treat a neoplasm in 21-28 days by changing the malignant anaerobic metabolism and the aerobic metabolism, which will thus become a suitable environment for the repair of nucleotides altered by the toxic carcinogen?

One of the variants of this solution is left in the care of pharmacologists regarding the incorporation of deficient enzymes in the neoplastic tissue with the help of targeted liposomes.

Another option would be to perform experiments in the laboratory on mammals regarding the effect of adaptation to hypobaric hypoxia corresponding to an altitude of 6000 m, in parallel with ensuring an adequate anticancer diet presented above and the application of negative aeronautical sessions in concentrations corresponding to this altitude. , with step-by-step adjustment by repeated exposures, starting with 5-minute sessions and then increasing by 5 minutes each session, up to 120 minutes, after which it will gradually return to normal.

This practical proposal based on the biochemical processes that take place in the human body during the adaptation of the organism to blood and tissue level to hypobaric hypoxia could then be explained in patients with malignant diseases who still have preserved their cardiovascular functions to quasi-normal parameters. It is known that in a healthy adult the volume of O2 that can be transported by hemoglobin in 100 ml of blood is 20 ml of O2. The maximum volume of expired O2 that is fixed by 100 ml of blood is called the oxy-phonetic value and is between 18-22.

Oxy-euphoric power varies in some pathological conditions or physiological conditions (pregnancy). The degree of combination of Hb with O2 as well as the dissociation of oxyhemoglobin with the release of O2 is strongly

influenced by the partial pressure of oxygen in the external and tissue environment. O2 fixation on Hb takes place in the lungs where the partial pressure of O2 is higher (100 mmHg) and relatively higher pH, which allows Hb saturation with O2 in a proportion of 96%. Inside tissues where the partial pressure of O2 is lower (45 mmHg) and lower pH due to the higher concentration of CO2, the end product of the citric cycle, some of which is in the form of ionized carbonic acid, oxyhemoglobin dissociates with the release of O2 which diffuses into tissues and becomes available for cellular respiration.

We notice that at the O2 pressure in the tissues, the hemoglobin remains saturated with O2 in a proportion of 65%. The difference of 30% is the amount of O2 given to the tissues. The sigmoidal aspect of the Hb saturation curve with O2 as a function of the O2 partial pressure as well as that of the oxyhemoglobin dissociation curves at different CO2 partial pressures shows that at low oxygen pressures Hb oxygenation takes place at first very slowly because then to grow fast. This is characteristic of allosteric curves.

Everything happens as if the fixation of a subunit molecule of the Hb molecule changes its shape and with it, the interaction between subunits, increases the affinity of the other subunits of Hb for O2. This phenomenon, known as the cooperative effect or cooperativity, is of great physiological importance because, at the partial pressure of oxygen of 35-45 mmHg existing in the tissues, the release of O2 from oxyhemoglobin occurs due to this particularity of the curve.

As the pH increases at an existing O2 partial pressure, the degree of saturation of Hb with O2 increases. This effect, as mentioned above, occurs in the lungs. Conversely, the decrease in pH due to the increase in the concentration of H ions, produced in the tissues by the passage of CO2 in the blood, hydration and dissociation of carbonic acid, increases the degree of dissociation of oxy-hemoglobin.

This reversible effect occurs because oxyhemoglobin being ionized for each bound O2 releases a proton:

H-Hb + O2 Hb…….> O2 + H +, wherein H-Hb + represents the protonated form of a reduced Hb substance. As this reaction is reversible, the increase in H + ion concentration causes the equilibrium to shift to the left (decreases the degree of oxyhemoglobin formation), while the decrease in H + concentration causes the equilibrium to shift to the right (increasing the degree of Hb saturation with O2).

This effect of pH on the O2 + Hb......> Hb O2 equilibrium is known under the name Bohr effect. The explanation of the phenomenon of cooperativity of Hb substances as well as of the Bohr effect was given by Perutz based on the conformational changes of Hb. In addition to the sigmoidal aspect of the Hb saturation curve with O2 and the influence of CO2 (via pH) on the transport of O2 in erythrocytes, another compound is formed, 2.3 di-phospho-glyceric acid (DPG) which exerts an important effect on Hb oxygenation. The Hb oxygenation process begins with chain 1 followed by chain 2, followed by the release of DPG and the oxygenation of chains B1 and B2.

In deoxygenated Hb all Hb bonds are broken, DPG is released and thyroxine residues are expelled into hydrophobic pockets. Hb oxygenation is therefore a gradual process, which explains the sigmoidal aspect of the oxygenation curve by increasing the affinity of Hb subunits for O2 as the assurance continues. The Bohr effect can be explained by changing the ionization constants of groups that form saline bonds in Hb but are free in oxyhemoglobin.

Adaptation and compensation mechanisms can, up to a point, provide partial values of compatible intracellular O2 pressure as normal activity at this level, even if Pa O2 values deviate far from normal. The existing O2 deficiency at an altitude of over 6000-7000 m determines, even in the state of physical rest, respiration with alveolar hyperventilation that leads to the elimination by way of expired air, excessively CO2. As a result, the non-gaseous alkaline composition will predominate in the blood, with bicarbonate causing alkalosis.

Alkalosis at height is partially offset by the fact that in the absence of O2 in expired air, the metabolism in the body is anaerobic. Metabolic anaerobic products have an acidic reaction by reacting with bicarbonate. Alkalosis, regardless of how it is produced, respiratory or metabolic, combines two stages:

I. The first stage, compensated alkalosis, in which the ratio does not change, changes only the absolute amount of bicarbonate or carbonic acid, such as respiratory or metabolic alkalosis.

II. Alkalosis becomes compensated when the bicarbonate / carbonic acid ratio changes, rising above 20 when the blood pH rises. We recall that at a partial O2 pressure of 100-150mmHg, Hb in the blood saturates with O2 turning into oxyhemoglobin. Here are the partial pressures of oxygen as a

function of altitude and the effect of the hypoxic, hypobaric environment on the saturation of hemoglobin with O_2:

• At atmospheric pressure with: (barometric, 760 mmHg) - pa O_2 in air = 159 mmHg, => - pa O_2 in alveoli = 104 mmHg - pa CO_2 in the alveoli = 50 mmHg. - Hb saturation with O_2 = 97%.

• At atmospheric pressure with: (at an altitude of 3000 m which is 547 mmHg) - pa O_2 in air = 110 mmHg, => - pa O_2 in the alveolus = 76 mmHg - pa CO_2 in the alveolus = 36 mmHg. - Hb saturation with O_2 = 90%.

• At atmospheric pressure with corresponding other. 6000 m (which is 349 mmHg) - pa O_2 in air = 73 mmHg - pa O_2 in the alveolus = 40 mmHg - pa CO_2 in the alveolus = 24 mmHg - Hb saturation in O_2 = 70%.

Hypoxia will cause a decrease in tissue O_2 tension that is related to cellular oxidation. As the partial blood pressure of O_2 decreases, Hb will contain less and less O_2. The appearance of the state of cyanosis indicates in all cases significant capillary hypoxia, discharging more than 30-40% of O_2 from oxyhemoglobin. Respiratory failure can occur in people suffering when O_2 drops below 60 mmHg (8 K Pa).

The normal values of pa O_2 according to age are 100-96 mmHg (13.3 - 12.8 KPa) for the ages of 20-30 years and 83-79 mmHg (11.0 - 10.5 KPa) for the ages of 60-70 years. Decreasing the O_2 partial pressure by half the normal value, ie to 50 mmHg, decreases by only 5-6 per cent the O_2 saturation of Hb, whereas at low partial pressures the release of O_2 is done quickly.

This behavior promotes the attachment of O_2 in the blood to the lungs and its release into the tissues. The difference (gradient) between the O_2 partial pressure in the arterioles blood and that inside the cells varies with the intensity of the metabolic processes on which the local use of O_2 depends. Thus, at the level of redox mitochondrial crystals (home of enzymes), the partial pressure of O_2 can drop below 1 mmHg, achieving a gradient of 89 mmHg compared to Pa O_2 of 90 mmHg (in the normal subject).

The amount of O_2 provided by cellular metabolic processes per unit of time depends in addition to this gradient and the proper functioning of the lungs. Once inside the O_2 cells, it is mostly used as the final acceptor of electrons from a long chain of oxidative degradation reactions of energy-generating substances.

In summary, we state that organic food substances are degraded in the body during a series of hydration, decarboxylation, etc. reactions, which transform complex molecules into increasingly simple molecules, simultaneously releasing energy, used in synthesis processes and in those that ensure the normal development of the functions of the various tissues and organs. Energy release is the result of enzyme-catalyzed exergonic reactions. During these reactions, the (e-) hydrogen electron is transformed step by step into respiratory.

Glycolysis in malignant cells:

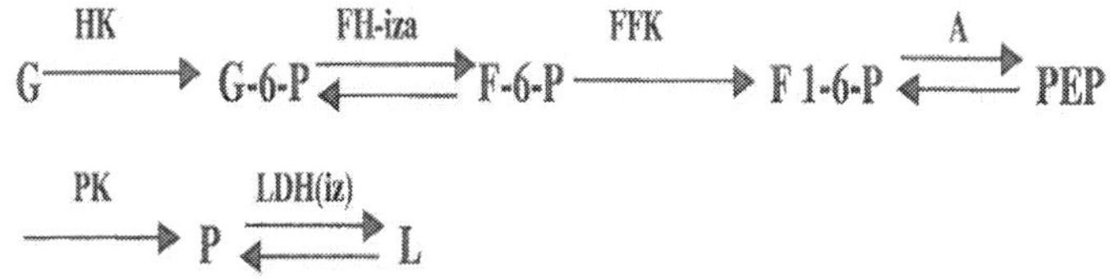

Last option, namely that initially the cellular infrastructures, would be damaged by toxic factors, infectious or permanent, even in small but cumulative doses. As oncogenes are older due to phylogeny, they may be the last to withstand aggression. The discovery of Peyton Rous at the turn of the century, the virus that causes bird sarcoma, was the first confirmation of the viral hypothesis behind cancer. Protein phosphorylation is known to be a normal process in cell metabolism. The synthesis of phosphorylated proteins with enzymatic characters is determined by a group of genes called normal proto-oncogenic cells. Several such genes have been isolated, stating that they are involved in the development of the cell cycle by regulating the multiplication and differentiation or maturation of cells.

Since basic sequences similar to those in proto-oncogenes have been found in simple life forms, they are considered to be very old and therefore essential for life.

Their transformation into oncogenes is possible in two ways:

1) By structural mutation when the products it encodes become normal;

2) By exaggerated multiplication or excessive activity with elaboration in large quantities of products that intervene in the cellular metabolism.

Recent genetic research has revealed genes with an inhibitory role: antioncogenes. Because their exact location is unknown, these progenitor

antagonists have been called suppressor genes. There are genes that, if inactivated or disrupted, are prone to cancer. There is a double system in which excessive activation of stimulant genes is as harmful as the inactivation of inhibitory genes.

After the 1970s, the possibility of cancer was highlighted by altering the genetic structures, respectively the DNA in the nucleus. It is necessary to combine two factors: genetic predisposition and exogenous toxins. These toxins can be mutagenic clinical substances, ionizing radiation, viruses, etc. Simply put, malignant tissue appears as a disorder of cell proliferation and maturation that results in completely normal shapes, structures, and functions.

Structurally distorted, malignant cells escape the control of the body, and become autonomous, multiplying infinitely without ever maturing until death. In the form of proto-oncogenes, they control proliferation and differentiation (maturation) but by the transformation they become carcinogenic.

Several explanations have been found in this regard:

• localized mutations;

• changing a base in the structure of DNA with the introduction of other amino acids in the products produced.

Consequent, these products of the respective genes are either functionally blocked or partially modified;

• amplifying the number of copies of a gene. This mechanism has been found in colon cancer;

• the movement of a proto-oncogene in the vicinity of an intensely active gene; for example, immunoglobulin genes in lymphoid cells;

• translocation, dislocation, rupture of a portion of two non-homologous chromosomes followed by reciprocal exchange of segments;

• introduction of an abnormal portion into a proto-oncogene. Suppressor genes slow down the transcription of their progenitors and exert an opposite effect on the target molecules at which the transcription of genetic information into a messenger ribonucleic acid for specific protein synthesis occurs.

It was known beforehand that the replacement of a defective chromosome stops the malignancy of the cell. This suggests that the malignant cell has one or more defective genes that are essential for a normal life. The loss of inhibitory genetic information is as harmful as the over-function of oncogenes that stimulate cell proliferation.

The presence of suppressor genes has been accurately detected at the chromosomal level. For cancer to occur, both the suppressor gene inherited from the father and the mother must be altered. In the case of a single gene failure, there is only one predisposition. Here are some chromosomal deficiencies found in some human tumors: • lung cancer, Cr 3 p (p = short arm)

• rectal cancer, Cr 3 p

• breast cancer, Cr 11 p

• colon cancer, Cr 17 p

• LGC cancer, LA = Cr 9 q (q = long arm)

• retinoblastoma cancer, Cr 13 q

• gastric cancer, Cr 13 q

• neuroblastoma cancer, Cr 1 p

• meningioma cancer, Cr 22 q

In other words, where the individual inherits both defective suppressor genes, from mother and father, endogenous cancer is established, and if the inherited genetic defect is restricted to only one suppressor gene, carcinogenesis is established under the influence of toxic, chemical, and physical factors, infectious, **[Figure 6].**

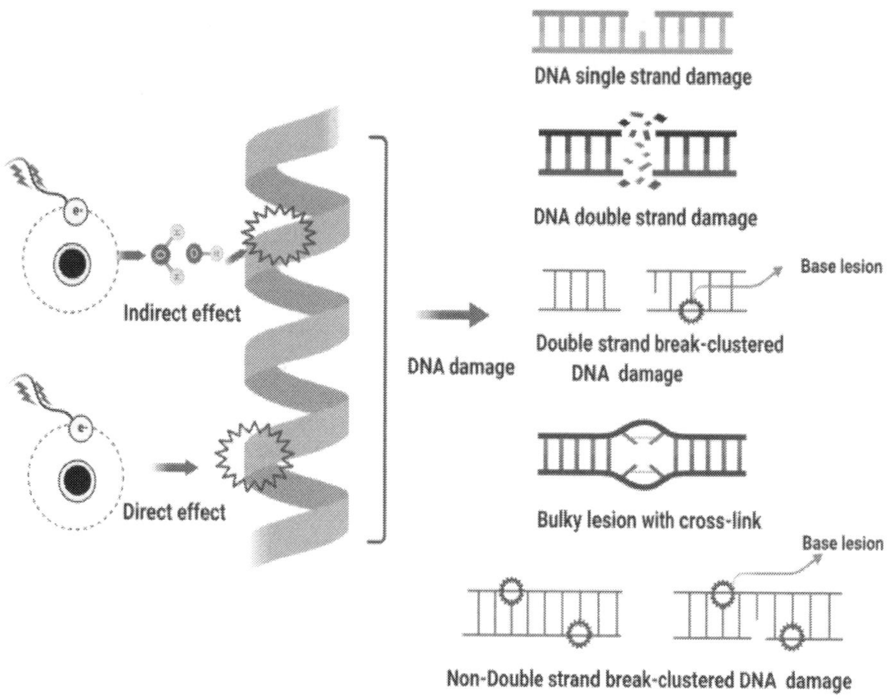

Figure 6. F*actors, especially certain environmental hazards such as toxic heavy metals and ionizing radiation, have been intensively studied and found to cause serious DNA damage*

The suppressor genes can also be altered by viruses, which has been shown not only in viruses well known as malignant in vitro, such as adenoviruses but also in some benign ones belonging to the herpes group (involvement of Epstein-Barr virus in nasopharyngeal cancer).

Whyte et al, 1995, discovered in the adenovirus the E1A gene responsible for malignant cells in mammals. These viruses malign not only by modifying the suppressor gene but also by blocking its product, which is equivalent to altering the genes. For example, the carcinogenic adenovirus synthesizes a complex of three cellular proteins, of which E1A is a protein identical to the product developed by the Rb genes. The Rb gene encodes a phosphoprotein that locates in the nucleus to bind to DNA. This phosphoprotein limits cell proliferation in both the retina and other tissues. Alteration of the Rb gene is a key factor in the onset of retinoblastoma.

Wilms tumor (embryonic carcinoma of the kidney) is caused by alteration of the 11q13 genes and the introduction of the normal chromosome 11 into the cells prevents the appearance of the neoplasm. In meningioma, the lack of a suppressor gene was found on the long arm of chromosome 22, the benignity being explained by the loss of a single copy of the gene. This situation was found in acoustic neurinoma in which a suppressor gene suffers.

Given these aspects, we can conclude that proto-oncogenes become oncogenic through structural changes and non-physiological activations under conditions of inadequate anaerobic metabolism. Inhibitory suppressor genes whose absence or inactivation due to their damage or non-expression in the metabolic conditions created by chronic cellular suffering at some point generate this disorder.

Substitution of normal proteins normally produced by suppressor genes or the creation of metabolic conditions for the physiological repair of damaged genes would be physiological antitumor procedures without side effects that would oppose uncontrolled tumor proliferation.

It is believed that in the process of carcinogenesis, the mitochondria of normal cells would be attacked by carcinogens and partially damaged, and the DNA would be better protected by the double nuclear membrane. Suppressor gene damage would occur later than mitochondrial damage. Subsequently, the nuclear barriers will give way and the DNA will be functionally damaged (carcinogenesis) or physically damaged (cancer installed) by reactivating oncogenes that find their natural environment of expression in a phylogenetic-scale anaerobic environment similar to the primary one.

If the cell were permanently restored to its original state of aerobiosis by the cessation of toxic factors, the cell could find the potential to repair its DNA through its enzymes, especially DNA ligase with the participation of ATP.

The importance of DNA in the development of vital processes both as a structural element, chromosomal and functional component, preservation and transmission of genetic information, and protein biosynthesis justifies the consideration of this component as the ultimate main target of toxic, physical, chemical, biological factors in general and radiation ionic in particular. Viral factors induce mutations or express cellular oncogene by insertion into cell DNA with gene dislocation or nuclear hybridization. The structural changes that radiation produces in DNA in the cellular context

may explain the obvious macroscopic effects, biochemical and genetic functional disturbances, and even cell death.

The energy required to induce a single single-chain rupture in mammals is 50 eV-100 eV if it was done in an oxygen atmosphere. The irradiated cell can recover by removing sublethal lesions. Experiments have shown that the potentially lethal lesion in the cell can be altered or converted by changing environmental conditions immediately after irradiation.

This phenomenon has been called cell restoration or restoration. The repair mechanisms consist of completing the rupture ("gap") caused by an enzymatic excision and each of them contains several stages of reaction: the separatory replication, the phenomenon of "defect of replicative synthesis" of DNA and the reunion of the strands that will eventually lead to the restoration of the contents of the broken polynucleotide chain. These processes are catalyzed by pre-existing enzymes in the cells, enzymes that promptly intervene in the recognition and repair of the lesion. Of these, the DNA ligase that acts for the act is deliberately detached.

It is known that 228 kcal and redox potential of about 10 eV arise from the Krebs cycle coupled with oxidative phosphorylation. If 50-100 eV from radiation is added to this potential, it means that the sum of the accumulated energy becomes harmful to the mitochondria and the cell nucleus. This harmful overload could also explain the cellular metabolic overload with destructive effects due to the very high rate of catabolism of superstructures in the body's stresses.

High aerobic metabolism at high parameters eventually leads to the installation of anaerobic metabolism. The aerobic change in anaerobic metabolism was observed by the Japanese in altitude adaptation experiments. Exposure to hypobaric hypoxia corresponding to an altitude above 6000 m initially causes, before the adaptation of the organism, a decrease of the ATP reserve and an increase of cAMP that will activate more intensely phosphofructokinase.

A marked increase in lactate and uric acid in exposure above 6000 m indicates that glycolysis is essential and that the aerobic metabolism of fatty acids is not essential for the generation of ATP in tissues in the acute phase of exposure of the non-acclimatized organism. Exposure to a high hypoxic altitude causes a metabolic and biochemical change and causes a change in the concentration of O2 in the blood and tissues. Once the adaptation is made, there is a stimulation of the oxidative metabolism given by the

intensification of the use of O2 in the mitochondria from the cellular oxygen reserves. Then there is the change in the ATP-forming reaction of anaerobic glycolysis to oxidative metabolism.

These results suggest that metabolic acclimatization to hypobaric hypoxia by repeated exposure at progressive altitudes up to 6000 m induces a change in energy metabolism from anaerobic glycolysis in the pre-adaptation period to aerobic metabolism when adaptation has been made. Returning to a normal altitude, this increased functional capacity of all cells in the body is maintained for a maximum of 21-28 days, after which the cellular parameters return to the previous normal forms. Can we treat a neoplasm in 21-28 days by changing the malignant anaerobic metabolism and the aerobic metabolism, which will thus become a suitable environment for the repair of nucleotides altered by the toxic carcinogen?

One of the variants of this solution is left in the care of pharmacologists regarding the incorporation of deficient enzymes in the neoplastic tissue with the help of targeted liposomes.

Another option would be to perform experiments in the laboratory on mammals regarding the effect of adaptation to hypobaric hypoxia corresponding to an altitude of 6000 m, in parallel with ensuring an adequate anticancer diet presented above and the application of negative aeronautical sessions in concentrations corresponding to this altitude. , with step-by-step adjustment by repeated exposures, starting with 5-minute sessions and then increasing by 5 minutes each session, up to 120 minutes, after which it will gradually return to normal.

This practical proposal based on the biochemical processes that take place in the human body during the adaptation of the organism to blood and tissue level to hypobaric hypoxia could then be explained in patients with malignant diseases who still have preserved their cardiovascular functions to quasi-normal parameters. It is known that in a healthy adult the volume of O2 that can be transported by hemoglobin in 100 ml of blood is 20 ml of O2. The maximum volume of expired O2 that is fixed by 100 ml of blood is called the oxy-phonetic value and is between 18-22.

Oxy-euphoric power varies in some pathological conditions or physiological conditions (pregnancy). The degree of combination of Hb with O2 as well as the dissociation of oxyhemoglobin with the release of O2 is strongly influenced by the partial pressure of oxygen in the external and tissue environment. O2 fixation on Hb takes place in the lungs where the partial

pressure of O2 is higher (100 mmHg) and relatively higher pH, which allows Hb saturation with O2 in a proportion of 96%. Inside tissues where the partial pressure of O2 is lower (45 mmHg) and lower pH due to the higher concentration of CO2, the end product of the citric cycle, some of which is in the form of ionized carbonic acid, oxyhemoglobin dissociates with the release of O2 which diffuses into tissues and becomes available for cellular respiration.

We notice that at the O2 pressure in the tissues, the hemoglobin remains saturated with O2 in a proportion of 65%. The difference of 30% is the amount of O2 given to the tissues. The sigmoidal aspect of the Hb saturation curve with O2 as a function of the O2 partial pressure as well as that of the oxyhemoglobin dissociation curves at different CO2 partial pressures shows that at low oxygen pressures Hb oxygenation takes place at first very slowly because then to grow fast. This is characteristic of allosteric curves.

Everything happens as if the fixation of a subunit molecule of the Hb molecule changes its shape and with it, the interaction between subunits, increases the affinity of the other subunits of Hb for O2. This phenomenon, known as the cooperative effect or cooperativity, is of great physiological importance because, at the partial pressure of oxygen of 35-45 mmHg existing in the tissues, the release of O2 from oxyhemoglobin occurs due to this particularity of the curve.

As the pH increases at an existing O2 partial pressure, the degree of saturation of Hb with O2 increases. This effect, as mentioned above, occurs in the lungs. Conversely, the decrease in pH due to the increase in the concentration of H ions, produced in the tissues by the passage of CO2 in the blood, hydration and dissociation of carbonic acid, increases the degree of dissociation of oxy-hemoglobin.

This reversible effect occurs because oxyhemoglobin being ionized for each bound O2 releases a proton:

H-Hb + O2 Hb> O2 + H +, wherein H-Hb + represents the protonated form of a reduced Hb substance. As this reaction is reversible, the increase in H + ion concentration causes the equilibrium to shift to the left (decreases the degree of oxyhemoglobin formation), while the decrease in H + concentration causes the equilibrium to shift to the right (increasing the degree of Hb saturation with O2).

This effect of pH on the O2 + Hb......> Hb O2 equilibrium is known under the name Bohr effect. The explanation of the phenomenon of cooperativity

of Hb substances as well as of the Bohr effect was given by Perutz based on the conformational changes of Hb. In addition to the sigmoidal aspect of the Hb saturation curve with O2 and the influence of CO2 (via pH) on the transport of O2 in erythrocytes, another compound is formed, 2.3 di-phospho-glyceric acid (DPG) which exerts an important effect on Hb oxygenation. The Hb oxygenation process begins with chain 1 followed by chain 2, followed by the release of DPG and the oxygenation of chains B1 and B2.

In deoxygenated Hb all Hb bonds are broken, DPG is released and thyroxine residues are expelled into hydrophobic pockets. Hb oxygenation is therefore a gradual process, which explains the sigmoidal aspect of the oxygenation curve by increasing the affinity of Hb subunits for O2 as the assurance continues. The Bohr effect can be explained by changing the ionization constants of groups that form saline bonds in Hb but are free in oxyhemoglobin.

Adaptation and compensation mechanisms can, up to a point, provide partial values of compatible intracellular O2 pressure as normal activity at this level, even if Pa O2 values deviate far from normal. The existing O2 deficiency at an altitude of over 6000-7000 m determines, even in the state of physical rest, respiration with alveolar hyperventilation that leads to the elimination by way of expired air, excessively CO2. As a result, the non-gaseous alkaline composition will predominate in the blood, with bicarbonate causing alkalosis.

Alkalosis at height is partially offset by the fact that in the absence of O2 in expired air, the metabolism in the body is anaerobic. Metabolic anaerobic products have an acidic reaction by reacting with bicarbonate. Alkalosis, regardless of how it is produced, respiratory or metabolic, combines two stages:

I. The first stage, compensated alkalosis, in which the ratio does not change, changes only the absolute amount of bicarbonate or carbonic acid, such as respiratory or metabolic alkalosis.

II. Alkalosis becomes compensated when the bicarbonate / carbonic acid ratio changes, rising above 20 when the blood pH rises. We recall that at a partial O2 pressure of 100-150mmHg, Hb in the blood saturates with O2 turning into oxyhemoglobin. Here are the partial pressures of oxygen as a function of altitude and the effect of the hypoxic, hypobaric environment on the saturation of hemoglobin with O2:

• At atmospheric pressure with: (barometric, 760 mmHg) - pa O2 in air = 159 mmHg, => - pa O2 in alveoli = 104 mmHg - pa CO2 in the alveoli = 50 mmHg. - Hb saturation with O2 = 97%.

• At atmospheric pressure with: (at an altitude of 3000 m which is 547 mmHg) - pa O2 in air = 110 mmHg, => - pa O2 in the alveolus = 76 mmHg - pa CO2 in the alveolus = 36 mmHg. - Hb saturation with O2 = 90%.

• At atmospheric pressure with corresponding other. 6000 m (which is 349 mmHg) - pa O2 in air = 73 mmHg - pa O2 in the alveolus = 40 mmHg - pa CO2 in the alveolus = 24 mmHg - Hb saturation in O2 = 70%.

Hypoxia will cause a decrease in tissue O2 tension that is related to cellular oxidation. As the partial blood pressure of O2 decreases, Hb will contain less and less O2. The appearance of the state of cyanosis indicates in all cases significant capillary hypoxia, discharging more than 30-40% of O2 from oxyhemoglobin. Respiratory failure can occur in people suffering when O2 drops below 60 mmHg (8 K Pa).

The normal values of pa O2 according to age are 100-96 mmHg (13.3 - 12.8 KPa) for the ages of 20-30 years and 83-79 mmHg (11.0 - 10.5 KPa) for the ages of 60-70 years. Decreasing the O2 partial pressure by half the normal value, ie to 50 mmHg, decreases by only 5-6 per cent the O2 saturation of Hb, whereas at low partial pressures the release of O2 is done quickly.

This behavior promotes the attachment of O2 in the blood to the lungs and its release into the tissues. The difference (gradient) between the O2 partial pressure in the arterioles blood and that inside the cells varies with the intensity of the metabolic processes on which the local use of O2 depends. Thus, at the level of redox mitochondrial crystals (home of enzymes), the partial pressure of O2 can drop below 1 mmHg, achieving a gradient of 89 mmHg compared to Pa O2 of 90 mmHg (in the normal subject).

The amount of O2 provided by cellular metabolic processes per unit of time depends in addition to this gradient and the proper functioning of the lungs. Once inside the O2 cells, it is mostly used as the final acceptor of electrons from a long chain of oxidative degradation reactions of energy-generating substances.

In summary, we state that organic food substances are degraded in the body during a series of hydration, decarboxylation, etc. reactions, which transform complex molecules into increasingly simple molecules, simultaneously releasing energy, used in synthesis processes and in those that ensure the

normal development of the functions of the various tissues and organs. Energy release is the result of enzyme-catalyzed exergonic reactions.

CHAPTER XI

ELECTROMAGNETIC GEO-COSMIC RADIATION, MODULATORS OF CELLULAR BIORHYTHMS

In the context of Eastern philosophies and the theory of modern quantum physics, TIME is the essence of the UNIVERSE, and the interior of the energy quantum (**photon Ef = hv**) also belongs to the essence of the Universe. It is assumed that TIME itself is organized in a positive, material, perceptible structure, as well as in a negative, imperceptible structure, as an energy sum, on its scale of degradation into insensitive vibrations, at the level of tangibility INFINIT - FINIT, in "Black-Holes" points.

According to the laws of classical physics, we have always relied on the notion of absolutely three-dimensional space, independent of the material things it contains and of an absolute time as a separate dimension and as constant energy, independent of the material world, (S = v x t) where S" is space, "v" is speed and "t" is time.

In more recent times, the theory of relativity has shown that space and time are intimately and inseparably linked, forming a four-dimensional continuum called:

ENERGY - SPACE - TIME - MATTER

Most unstable particles have an extremely short lifespan, less than one-millionth of a second. This means that the time of the Universe is NOT INFINITE because one second, (1 s\`), is born from 10^{24} eV, and the universe has innate **energy > 10^{31} eV / s. In the formula ENERGY-TIME-SPACE-LIGHT, any object is a form of light stopped in a mattery structure and the man is an accident of light.**

In the perceptible, visible way, the light turns into darkness, but at the imperceptible level the transformation of existence into light takes place through the emission of energetic radiation from the entire Universe, where the time of life photon is $10^{-15\ s}$ and the energy derivation is transformed into light-years (1 light-year = 75 million km/energy space): $t = \alpha / c = \alpha h$

/ E γ, (gamma (γ) energy)

In this way we can consider light as a prenatal state, as an unorganized time in a structure, which comes from infinity at the level of tangential INFINITY - FINITE, in the points of the "white holes" - WHITE - HOLES.

According to the formula $\alpha = c \times t$, an energy wave hv of 0.04 eV to become a light particle needs 0.33 x 10^{-15}s, during which time it will travel space of 10^{-7} m on a vacuum space of 10^{-7} m, (10^3 A) any electromagnetic energy wave in 10^{15} eV voltage can be transformed in minimum energy value of 0.04 eV as a material particle, becoming photon. This phenomenon also exists in the microcosm of the atom when an electron passes from the upper energy level to the lower energy layer. In the field theory of modern physics. The vid appears as a dynamic quantity of great importance. Because the reality behind all phenomena exceeds our possibilities of description, it is considered to be out of shape or empty, which does not mean that it is a wasteland. On the contrary, it is a vid with infinite creative potential.

The notion of physical vid, as it appears in field theory, contains the potential of all forms in the particle world. The idea of a universe that expands and contracts periodically involves a scale of time and space.

Descending on the scale of Space, in Time, the cosmic energy field is a quantum field, ex, a field that can take the form of quantum or particles E = hv. COSMIC RADIATION contains mass particles whose origin has not been elucidated, engaged in a continuous cosmic dance of ENERGY.

These particles are subject to a gravity field of 10^{12} eV. Man is given to be satisfied with the discontinuity of energetic perception of human structures, and although he is endowed with imperfect means of receiving the energetic vibrations of the Universe, he always aspires to comprehend the vibrations of the Cosmos from the undegraded world of INFINITY.

Infinity is the spatiality that has only the interior. A contemplation of infinity outside it is not possible. Concerning infinity, any object is internal and subject to its evolution. The degree of the interiority of the phenomenon to infinity determines the degree of the infinity of the phenomenon. This leads to the conclusion that everything is equal to something else in the pure essence of the quanta energy hv emanated from the ENTROPY of its existence.

The discovery that MASS is only a form of energy (E = mc2 / 2, and m = 2E / c2) implies that the nature of subatomic particles is intrinsically

dynamic and that its matter and activity are only different aspects of the same temporal space reality. In this way, all objects can be seen as processes of a universal energy flow.

The basic elements of the substance are dynamic patterns, transient stages in a constant process of transformation and change, and the properties of subatomic particles can only be understood in terms of motion, interaction, and transformation. SPACE and LIGHT represent a concrete form of TIME, a release of TIME into discontinuous, concrete energetic forms. The unification of TIME and SPACE implies an aspect: the existence of matter not can be separated from its activity in vibratory motion. Physics imagines its matter in a continuous dance with a condensation density of the hv energy quanta. The size of the condensation density determines the formation of new energies of lower energy, in a new stratification – LIGHT.

If in INFINITY, reality appears undivided and undifferentiated, on the huge scale of the UNIVERSE, gradually, the subatomic units of matter, as abstract entities, with a dual aspect of particles and where, unite in the infra-microscopic solid matter under the influence of intrinsic forces, and when they become a perfect structure to its extreme, they will gradually return to achieve the opposite.

In the known UNIVERSE, energy particles are subjected to fields of a very different nature: fields of temperature, pressure, deformation, voltage, electrical, magnetic, and nuclear, in each of these fields, force involves a movement in the evolution of a process. At the same time, non-living matter, at the microscopic or submicroscopic level, will have a life of its own, due to time shifts, and intrinsic chemical and structural defects. The energetic condensation of photons along cosmic forces means the transformation of LIGHT - MATTER:

Electronic super density at the same time implies a super density of "positive" opposite charges, which determines the formation of matter as an entity of internal oppositional bonds. Condensation of energy waves in the immediately lower layers gives rise to energy interactions that are reflected in the form of mass, called subatomic particles. The stronger the interactions, the greater the possibility of the phenomenon of exchange.

FORCE and MATTER have a common origin in these dynamic models called particles. Force, according to the theories of Eastern philosophies, as a harmony of the movement within things, resembles the modern theory in which the forces between particles reflect dynamic patterns inherent in these

particles.

From these energetic interactions arise mass particles with weak interaction: photons and leptons, and particles with strong interaction: electrons, protons and neutrons. Most of the particles will be strongly interacting and we will call them HADRONS. Photons, electrons and protons form stable particles, which will be annihilated only by collision, while the neutron disintegrates spontaneously, transforming into a proton accompanied by a created electron and a new massless particle, neutrino.

Neutrino is as stable as protons and electrons. There is also an antiparticle for each particle with equal mass, just the opposite charge. When the Cosmic Rays have higher energy, they hit the Earth's atmosphere, collide with waves in the atmosphere's molecules, and produce various secondary particles that either disintegrate or collide further until the last of them touches the Earth.

In this way, a single proton entering the Earth's atmosphere can give rise to a cascade of phenomena in which the initial kinetic energy is transformed into a rain of different particles and is gradually absorbed as they enter the ATMOSPHERE. According to the theory of energy conservation, all particle interactions are symmetric relative to the movement in TIME and SPACE.

Modern physics assumes that all hadrons are made up of a small number of entities - elements called quarks. It is accepted that all hadrons are composed of 3 types of quarks, and each quark appears in 3 varieties, designated for the colors: red, white, yellow, and blue, the colors of human esoteric fields.

Hadron reactions are a flow of energy in which particles are created and dissolved, but the energy in space can only flow through certain "channels" characterized by quantum numbers conserved in strong interactions.

Thus, the energy quantum in the antimatter-matter aggregate in the infrared cosmic field has an energy of 4×10^{-3} eV, and the energy quantum in the inert atomic-molecular aggregate in the galactic cosmic field has an energy of 4×10^{-7} eV, similar to the radio astronomy wave. In the "S-matrix" theory originally proposed by Heisenberg in 1943, which is a series of probabilities for all possible reactions in which hadrons are involved, the "reaction channel concept" is more important than the particle concept.

It is referred to as a set of quantum numbers that can be carried in a series of combinations of HADRONS, namely the combination of HADRONS,

strong particle-strong particle (protons), strong particle-weak particle (neutrons), strong particle-antiparticle, (quark-antiquark) with a weak particle final result is a matter of probability, which depends first on the amount of cosmic energy that is concentrated at a given time, on the time and space scale, measured in light-years (1 year- light = 70 million kilometers). All the particles are intermediate in a series of reactions.

The interaction forces of the electromagnetic waves in the cosmos are manifested as particles with a certain internal structure, whose mass determines the radius of force, the force being identified as an intrinsic property of the interacting particle (m = E / c 2). Nature cannot be reduced to fundamental entities such as elementary particles or fields, because the UNIVERSE is a dynamic web of interconnected phenomena. None of the properties of any particle in this energy web is fundamental, as they all derive from the properties of the other particles formed in the global constellation of their mutual interactions, from the structure of the entire web. In perpetual change, there is no room for a fixed fundamental entity because either party continues the other. The static equilibrium of living matter at a given time results from the macroscopic balancing of the outer field interface with its inner fields.

The complexity of the phenomenon arises from the interaction of dynamic inner forces with the forces resulting from the theme fields pressure, pressure, electromagnetic radiation and gravitational fields. In each material particle is thus born a field of stresses and deformations, specific and dependent on time, on the state in which the matter, plasma (ionized gases, fumes, gaseous phase, liquid, solid) is at a given moment:

1. Disaggregated energy cosmic field: $\lambda = 10^{-14}$ **m,** $v = 10^{22}$ **Hz,** $hv = 4 \times 10^{5}$ **eV - cosmic radiation;**

2. Aggregate energy field - **LIGHT:** $\lambda = 10^{-7}$ **m,** $v = 10^{15}$ **Hz,** $hv = 4 \times 10^{-2}$ **eV - light radiation;**

3. Aggregate matter-antimatter: $\lambda = 10^{-7}$ **m,** $v = 10^{14}$ **Hz,** $hv = 4 \times 10^{-3}$ **eV - infrared field;**

4. Solid - inert aggregate: $\lambda = 10^{-2}$ **m,** $v = 10^{10}$ **Hz,** $hv = 4 \times 10^{-7}$ **eV - astronomical waves;**

5. Viable molecular aggregate: $\lambda = 10^{-4}$ **m,** $v = 10^{4}$ **Hz,** $hv = 4 \times 10^{13}$ **eV - induction heating waves;**

6. Disaggregating energy field bio-magnetic: **$\lambda = 10^{-5}$ m, v = 10^{12} Hz, hv bio-energy 4 x 10^{-5} eV**.

At the same time, our natural environment in which we "swim", the air, could present in most samples, aspects of "interface" through the complex solid-air-solid, gas-air-gas, liquid-air-liquid connection, etc.

When a medium separates from another, for example, the delimitation in space of a solid field with the atmosphere and within the same geometric configuration, under the effect of internal and external fields, to which the non-living material is subjected, a resulting flow of particles, a train from where, due to electronic super density, energy field consists of energy particles called cotton - particles similar to tachyon particles, ex, with speeds higher than the speed of light (10 times the speed of light in a vacuum) and with a rest mass equal to zero, similar to photons, and which do not carry energy but which lead to a significant increase in internal energy, with the possibility of material structural changes.

These particles, with speeds higher than the speed of light, are emitted gradually, until the depletion of the material, specific to each material, raises the issue of "returning time" from the existence of the material from which they are emitted to the initial state of non-existence.

The density of matter in electrons is of the order of 10^{10} g / cm3. On a global, macroscopic scale, the average density of the planet is 5.51 t / m3, and the density of surface rocks is 2.5 t / m, which accredits the idea that high pressures and temperatures inside our planet cause a strong condensation of matter. At these densities the fields in the macrocosm emit waves.

The pulsars in the Sun have a density of 10^{6} - 10^{15} g / m3. The hypodensity in the microcosm of the atom would emit independent cations. The inanimate matter is amorphous, opaque and devoid of existential rhythm, instead, living matter, unitary with itself, in its entity, is a harmonious reverberation, of subtle, bio-magnetic energies, derived from the physic-chemical energies of its organs.

The inner energy of the being, trained in its vital arc, unfolded in a concrete and ephemeral time of the year, at the level of cellular nucleic acids and in the landscape of its own body, transmitted successively in the restructuring of its matter, can be argued and mirrored successively until COSMOS, on the path of information channels, invisible and insensitive, cell-cell, living molecule-dead molecule, inert matter-infinity-vacuum. The hv energy quanta derived from the aerobic and anaerobic degradation metabolisms

carry an energy of 4×10^{-13} eV similar to induction heating waves.

At the level of living matter, there is an interface of the exoteric, cosmic energies with the exoteric ones that derive from the manifestation of the vacuum, as an embodiment of the Divine Universal force. All living or non-living matter has a common denominator, the atom, the fundamental brick of matter. In fact, on Earth, living and non-living, with the elements of living-non-living transition, unexplained by science, intertwine harmoniously because at the molecular level plant biosensors - cellular receptors are common Physic-chemical elements in the mechanisms of reception of various forms of energy. environment.

At the level of the cerebral cortex, it has been observed that the distribution of neural "hot spots" in the passage of thought is very different depending on the speed of neural circuit connections in natural energy conversion systems and biosystems of transmission and processing of information reflected in consciousness. At the level of the psyche, an atomic pulverization of consciousness can take place over time. The ego's consciousness can also acquire huge powers that transcend spatiality and temporality, overcoming any inertia but which can also suffer potential drops depending on the astral biorhythm (diurnal-nocturnal, lunar-multiannual cycle) becoming at some point transiently captive, devoid of at the subconscious level of self-freedom.

If the undulating amplitude of endothermic bio-energies depends at some point on the influence of astral, exoteric energies, the rhythm of these energies belongs to thought, which with its intrinsic psychic force, unexplained by science, can lend, to a point, material forms of electromagnetic energy. from its bioenergetic organization, because things in the world themselves do not seem to know movement and growth towards an intelligible structure.

The intensity of the magnetic field of the brain was measured at the value of 1×10^3 Oe = 100 mT, compared to the intensity of the magnetic field of an ordinary living cell in the living body which rises to the value of 25 - 100 ft. I have in me the germinal power, which I can create precisely because of its inner relation to infinity, but the intensity of its bioenergy is different depending on its degree of interiority, that is, its ability to encompass its infinity by relating to it, feeling that is contained in it.

From the inner movements of the ego, from the energetic reverberations of the dominant neural circuits at a given moment, is born through the external

projection at the level of the afferent pathways, which is directed by the will of volition, an outer, endothermic, discontinuous externalization of the living, derived from the physicochemical processes of intermediate metabolic processing.

In this way, the outside world is forced to bow to the will to lucidly explore a self that, according to the imperious impulses of the being, remains violated in the entropic accounts. The frenetic urge to assert the ego in an outer universe is reflected in its inner things. In them, the thought of the Self, at the end of the targeted concentration, can appear as a definitive human conclusion.

Practically all biomaterial represents the dielectric placed between heaven and earth through which a continuous exchange of pulsating energy takes place, springing from its creation and the destruction of the perfection of the living organization on a microscopic and submicroscopic scale contained in the vibrations of the cosmos descending from the ungraded light of infinity.

The disaggregating energy field of the living human body was calculated at the value of 4x 10^5eV (0.04 mV) representing waves in the field of thermal radiation in the infrared-ultra-red field with v of 10^{12} Hz and λ of 10^{-4} m. The technology for measuring human bioenergy, springing from magnetic passes performed on experimental fluids was based on the accuracy, sensitivity and reproducibility of a digital pH-meter PH-MEHLER-6.32, Methrom, and the electrical and electromagnetic conversion was performed by mathematical calculations, {**Table 1**}.

Solutions under biomagnetic waves	**Initial pH**	**Bioenergetic pH**	**U(mV) inițial**	**U(mV) Bioenergetic**
Distilled H 2 O	7,11	7,82	-0,0187	-0,0620
NaCl 0,9% Solution	6,66	7,45	0,019	-0,025
Na_2CO_3 8% Solution	8,12	8,18	-0,063	0,067
Human Serum	7,45	7,51	-0,025	-0,019
Sol. buffer	7,00	7,08	0,000	-0,040

Table 1. Average energy values of bio-magnetised liquids of 100 experiments, using a device Ph-Meter for measurement changes of pH

Bioenergetic particle mass: **Mb** = $2 \times 4 \times 10^{-5} \times 1.6 \times 10^{-19} \times 10^{-7} \times 10^{-6} = 10^{-32}$ kg, approximately equal to 1/10 of the mass of the electron. Based on the phenomena of classical physics I = U / R and 1 Oe = 79.6 A / m, the intensity of the peripheral bioenergetic field of the upper limbs was calculated at 25 nT while the intensity of the bio-magnetic field of the entire cerebral cortex amounts to 100 mT (where each neuron has a magnetic field of 25 Ft).

The process of calculating the conversion of energy into seconds Starting from the classical formula of distance, S = v x t1 the relativistic formula of space becomes a = c x t, where c = the speed of light in a vacuum; t = photon decay time, calculated at 10^{-15} sec, with the wavelength of the photon of 10 -7 m; t = α / c = 10 -7 / (3 x10^{-9}) = 0.3 x 10^{-15} sec. Knowing the energy of the 0.04 eV photon, we can calculate the time in which this energy is created according to the relativistic formula:

Energy photon = αh /tγ, (γ=lamda)

If the energy of 0.04 eV occurs in 1.6 x 10^{-27} seconds and means that 25 x 10^{-24} eV will occur in one second. The potential of 25 x 1024 eV, which represents an energy state born from infinity, can be converted into the terrestrial unit of time, one second. This means that from 10^{31} eV / s, the universal energy, 1024 eV are transformed into second-time, and 10 7 eV into other forms of energy. Over time, 1024 eV transforms light years into space 10^{15} eV and space turns into the matter, with less than 10^{7} eV energy,

[Table 2].

Variables Energetic	Time – Space constants
Es = α h / t γ = Energy - Time - Space - Light	Time - life of photon = 10^{-15}s
The energy of a second Es = 25 x 10^{-24} eV	Universe time 7 x 10^{15} light-years
Photon energy Ef = 0.04 eV	Number of light years 10^{16}
Energy magnitude Einstein 11,97 x 10^{4} / γ γ = 10^{-14} – 10^{-7} m	Distance in energy space = 75 x 10^{9}/ m
The energy of the universe 3 x 10^{19} erg=2x10^{31} eV/s	Product = Universe Time x Photon Time = = 7 x 10^{15} x 10^{-15}=7
One year of light energy = 7 x 10^{15} eV	Product = Universe Time x Photon Time = 7 x 10^{15} x 10^{-15}=7
The energy of a calendar year 75 x 10^{31} eV	Photon frequency = 10^{15} Hz

Calculation parameters:

$t = \alpha / c = \alpha h / E \gamma$
$\alpha = t \times c$, where $c = 3 \times 10^8$ m/s
$h = 6{,}55 \times 10^{-27}$ erg/cm/s, where h – Constant Planck
1 erg = 10^{-7} J
1 eV = $1{,}6 \times 10^{-19}$ J
$\gamma f = 10^{-7}$ m
1 Gauss = 10 e = 10^{-1} mT = 1000/4τA/m
1 nT = 10^{-6} fT
1 Tesla = 1 Wb/m^2
1 W = 1 Vs
Electric potential = V = W/A

The physiological implications of bioenergy transferred to other living cells could occur in the autocratic system based on successive energy accumulations on the chromo-morphic groups in the cytochrome system, where the electron transport is done with EO between 0.04 - 0.27 eV, (40-270 mV).

-3e
$Fe\ Fe^{+++} + 3e^-$ ⟶

$2H^+ + 2Fe^{+++} H_2 + 2Fe^{+++}$ ⟶

This research has shown that by transforming raw chemical energy into a more subtle one, the great potential latent energy reserve that inhabits man can be released and used for beneficial purposes, in regulating cell physiology, without changes in the condition of visible matter emitting energies other than accompanying caloric energy. Bio-magnetic radiation that can be emitted by all living cells in the animal and plant kingdoms, as well as from metals, has been called "N" radiation by French researchers. Lifeless bodies, treated with chloroform, never emit such radiation, which proves that this bioenergy is constructive and coordinates physical molecules, cells, etc., and brings them together in a well-defined organism.

This bioenergy is a part of the universal breath of life that the human body acquires during the short time that we call "a life." Without it, the body would be at most a bunch of independent cells. This energy associates the cells into a whole, unique and complex, passing through the branches and meshes of the "vital network" - this brilliant and gilded network of unimaginable finesse, of delicate beauty, in the meshes of which the atoms are placed.

If we compare the astral energy values with the values of complementary human bio-genesis we can conclude that infinity is the reservoir of vital force. From infinity emanate the vital currents that vibrate through space as through the body of any living thing on earth. The whole microcosm is potentially contained in the "liquor vitae" "a nervous fluid ... in which the nature, quality, character and essence of all beings are found" (Paracelsus). Physically, this bioenergy is the controlling agent of all the chemical-physiological transformations in the protoplasm; it is the one that causes the differentiation and formation of different vegetal, and animal tissues, [10].

2. Electromagnetic, geo-cosmic radiation, modulators of cellular biorhythms

The earth was formed 4 billion years ago from dust and gas, with dust containing radioactive elements. Biological evolution was preceded by chemical evolution that lasted almost 1/3 of the earth's history. Solar energy in the form of radiation or electrical discharges was the primary source for the synthesis of molecules and even for polymerization, which led to biological molecules.

Endogenous cell rhythms were formed under the influence of environmental factors, later being fixed in the genome as independent rhythms ("congenital matrix"), which then suffer the influence of conformational change modelled under the action of environmental factors.

The Sun's 22-year magnetic cycle introduced 22-year periodicities in the variation of solar active phenomena in the parameters of the interplanetary magnetic field, geomagnetic activity and some meteo-climatic factors. A periodicity of about 2 years was highlighted in the intensity of galactic cosmic radiation and the characteristics of the solar wind and the indices of geomagnetic activity (Djapiashuili, 1982).

At total lunar eclipses, there was an increase in geomagnetic activity for four days (three days before and on the day of the eclipse). In solar eclipses, an intensification of geomagnetic activity occurs a few hours before the optical eclipse, and oscillations of ionospheric parameters are generated during the eclipse. Organisms are usually exposed to magnetic disturbances between sunrise and sunset. Outside the diurnal cycle of light, diurnal oscillations of the Earth's magnetic field support circadian biorhythms. At the heart of our concerns are cellular metal oscillations under the influence of magnetism and electromagnetism quantified in high-frequency biorhythms.

Periodic astronomical and geomagnetic phenomena with high frequencies similar to biological rhythms can be summarized as follows:

• Plasma electromagnetic waves with v = O, Hz-1 MHz;

• Geomagnetic pulses with v = 1-100 Hz. In solar flares, when magnetic storms occur, fluctuations between 5 Hz and tens of thousands of Hz occur;

• Regular-looking micro-pulses of the geomagnetic field with periods between 2.5-10 minutes (the most common being 5 minutes), with amplitude variations in the period over time. The appearance and amplitude of these pulses have a diurnal variation, with the maximum before noon (10.00). Micro-pulsation periods are minimal at 4.00.

The magnetic variations produced by the monthly tide have studied characteristics, the maximums being at 6.00 and 18.00 monthly time. The solar diurnal variation of the micro-pulsations of the geomagnetic field has a main minimum before noon. Earth-induced currents induced in the Earth's crust by variations in the atmospheric electromagnetic field and the geomagnetic field show periodicities in about 24 hours.

The interaction of the sectors of the interplanetary magnetic field with the Earth generates besides the period of 27-28 days and the subperiod of 12-14 days or 5-9 days in the variation of the intensity of the cosmic radiation and the geophysical parameters.

The variations of the geomagnetic flow induced by the Sun and the Moon are considered to influence the biochemical processes of the organism, especially in the CNS and the endocrine system and consequently determine changes in the development of biological rhythms. These variations influence the receptor areas of the body, namely the hypothalamus appreciated as a receptor of geomagnetic flux.

The intensity of the galactic cosmic radiation has a periodicity of 28 days, corresponding to the hormonal biorhythms. The Earth's magnetic field has a high in August-September and a low in January. From an astronomical point of view, it is estimated that the 11-year cycle highlighted by the evolution of solar phenomena represents an average value between the maximums and minimums of solar activity. Cosmic electromagnetic radiation of short wavelengths induces impulsive changes of about 500 nT in the horizontal component of the Earth's magnetic field (magnetic hooks).

Solar plasma emitted at high-velocity eruptions triggers high-intensity, sudden-onset magnetic storms, followed by rapid increases of one hundred of an nT of the horizontal component of the magnetic field. Before intense proton solar eruptions, there are disturbances precursors to eruptions of solar electromagnetic radiation, as well as in the ionospheric parameters and of the terrestrial magnetic field with intervals of more than 20 minutes (at X and UV radiation).

Pulses lasting about 20 minutes were also recorded in ionosphere parameters and geomagnetic activity at a total solar eclipse. The cell cycle, namely the DNA synthesis and mitosis phase, takes place at different times during the day. Thus, the rate of DNA synthesis (phase S) is placed around 18.00 while the mitosis phase (M) occurs it's around 4.00.

Cellular rhythms are dependent on synchronizers but especially on the endogenous impulses of the pacemaker, dictated by the genetic pacemaker. Thus, the intracellular processes are in phase with the frequency of the synchronizer that imposed the periodicity:

• Protein synthesis;

• Enzymatic reactions;

• VO2.

If there is a disagreement, the environment adjusts while the synchronizer is operating (altitude adjustments). Liver cell cultures were performed and the DNA content was determined before and after various treatments using a device called a cytopathic meter. It has been found that signals from phase G1 to phase S or the faster transaction from G0-G1 and G1-S can be influenced by circadian signals. It is known that the peak incorporation of thymidine H.3 corresponds to the time of DNA replication. The incorporation of thymidine with H3 corresponds to the variations in nuclease activity: during the dark period it is maximum, and the DNA turbine is minimal (and vice versa, during the day).

Within the high-frequency biorhythms with a period of up to 30 minutes we distinguish:

• Rhythms of enzymatic activity (aminotransferase, phosphatase) which are characterized by very high frequencies, respectively of the order of fractions of a second;

• Folding and twisting movements of DNA, which have a frequency of about one billion / S, with significance in the selective transmission of genetic information;

• Rhythms of nerve activity with alpha rhythms of 10 cycles / s. As part of the cell division cycle, the G1 standby phase is considered to be strictly unexpressed over time, while the S and G2 phases are invariant with time.

According to the probability model, after division the cell enters a phase in which its activity is not oriented towards G1 proliferation; the transition from phase G1 to phase S and then to G2 when DNA synthesis and mitosis take place, occurs with a certain probability at a certain time.

The factors listed above and several other factors, including magnetism, can speed up the cell's transition from standby to replication. Light affects the biological oscillator by opening membrane ion channels, which can be photosensitive or can be optically controlled by a photoreceptor. The circadian oscillatory function is relatively independent of the exact level of enzymatic activity. This independence of the clock mechanism from possible fluctuations in enzymatic activity is an adaptive advantage of the circadian "clock". Electromagnetic radiation whose energy is so low that they are unable to produce ionization of molecules, and therefore of biomolecules in biological systems, has been called non-ionized radiation. Their energy is placed below 10 eV and therefore they have a wavelength greater than 100 mm.

E = hv = hc — , where „c „ is light speed in vid

Exemplify, the ionization energy of carbon is 11.24 eV. The variation of the energy transmitted by the non-ionized radiations takes place according to the formula: E = Ee + Ev + Er where: Ee - represents the configuration energy of the electrons; Ev- is the vibrational energy of electrons; Er - rotational energy of electrons.

The excitation states of the transitional electrons are objectified into "singlet" ions, which have spins oriented antiparallel to the fundamental electrons. The excitation of these ions with the transition to the ground state is done by the remission of the photon absorbed from the "triplet" state by the phosphorescence phenomenon. These non-radioactive exciters will remove heat.

Radiation is not absorbed by the whole molecule but by certain groups in the molecule called chromophores: C = O -N = N C = C - N = O UV

radiation in the 240-290 nm range is absorbed by nucleic acids with the following effects:

• formation of dimers between pyrimidine bases;

• hydration of pyrimidine bases;

• breaking the H bonds;

• breaking DNA chains;

• formation of bonds with DNA proteins crosslinks.

These cellular traumas will delay or inhibit mitosis, and decrease the synthesis of proteins and nucleic acids while reducing respiratory exchanges. Microwaves are electromagnetic waves with a frequency between 300 - 300,000 MHz and a wavelength of 1 x 1O6 - 1 x 1O10 m. The intensity of the microwave field is measured in units of power W / cm2 for distances with a wavelength greater than the radiation source and A / cm2 for distances shorter than the wavelength.

Microwaves resonate and this is explained by the higher degree of absorption which is characteristic of biological materials. Their thermal effects mask other mechanisms of action. Ultrasound arises from the change in the size of a ferromagnetic body under the action of a magnetic field.

Under their influence, biological substances can be oxidized and polymerized. Ultrasound (US) breaks down nucleic acids, sulfuric acids, and hyaluronic acids. Proteins break down at peptide bonds, giving a combination of carbonyl and acid. Average intensities between 1 - 5 W / cm2 can lead to reversible cellular transformations marked by an acceleration of physiological phenomena.

High currents above 5 W / cm2 produce irreversible changes. The nuclei of the cells deform and lyse. Ionizing radiation: The human body is irradiated from the following sources of radiation: natural, sanitary, technical, and various. Natural irradiation is due to the natural background of radiation which consists of 30% cosmic radiation, 45% radiation from the activity of radio elements in the soil; 24% radiation of elements involved in metabolism and% radioactivity in the atmosphere. A man should not exceed 5 rem/year of natural irradiation. Water-soluble radiation protectors are usually substances that have NH2 and SH in their molecules.

R.1

-HS - (CH.2) – N -------

R.2

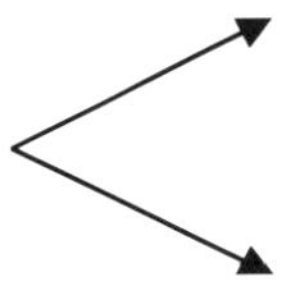

Various collaborators have suggested that the fluctuation of SH clusters that occurs in cell division may act as a mitotic clock. Such changes in the sulfhydryl groups are closely related to the synthesis of cleavage proteins. Under the action of ionizing radiation, macromolecules change their molecular weight, amino acids decarboxylate and rupture in peptide chains that break down and reconstitute. In other words, the colloidal substances can coagulate and the enzymes are inactivated to the greatest extent.

The ions resulting from this process can react with substances in the irradiated tissue, which determines the synthesis of new substances that disrupt normal physiological processes. The noticeable changes for proteins are given by radiation between 40-50 r / protein and go up to 2000-3000 r for fatty acids

Among the fat-soluble radioprotective substances are prostaglandins, hormones and various vitamins. Altering the stages of DNA biosynthesis leads to the birth of altered chromosomes that transmit abnormal characters to new cells. The alterations are mainly in the H-bridges in the DNA.

Depending on the intensity of the changes in chromosomes, structural changes may occur in some genes that may stimulate neoplastic processes or a wide range of mutations with immediate or delayed consequences, from a few seconds to several years. The effect of radiation is all the stronger as the cellular mitotic rate increases. The effect of irradiation is greater when the dose exceeds a certain threshold dose.

The need for natural irradiation for the development of organisms is discussed. Populations in regions with radioactive elements have gained radio-resistance. The physiological effects of small doses of natural radiation are located in the membrane, cytoplasm and nucleus. At the membrane level, low doses increase the permeability for ions, electrolytes, and the physiological oscillations of the resting potential of the cell membrane.

At the level of cytoplasm, it determines the modification of the osmotic resistance, the production of VO2 and the production of lactate. These

effects are good for a healthy body. The roentgenological system is used to measure the effects of X and γ radiation with energy up to 3 Me V. This system is based on measuring the ionization of the air by these radiations. X and γ radiation of 1.24 x 105 eV causes inhibition of cell division and the formation of free radicals. The energies of the particles emitted by radioactive nuclei range from about 0.1 to 10 MeV.

The total binding energy of the atomic nuclei is equal to the energy required to release all the particles in the nuclei. Particles are completely ionized helium nuclei. Disintegration is only valid for heavy cores. B radiation is the emission of electrons that arise from the decomposition of neutrons. In decay, the number of protons in the nucleus does not change (isomer nucleus).

The γ energy emitted represents the energy difference between two levels, excited and fundamental. In γ disintegration, the disintegration conditions are also known among light nuclei. At energies greater than 1 Me V, the transformation of γ radiation into an electron and positron causes dissociation and rupture of molecules, processes responsible for chemical, photo-dynamic and biological effects of radiation.

By emitting γ nuclei, the nuclei do not undergo a structural transformation but only a transition from one energetic state to another (isobaric nucleus). Nuclear decay is the tendency of physical systems to move to the lowest possible energy states. No one, not even the neighbor nucleus, knows when a nucleus disintegrates. There may be nuclei that disintegrate very late, others very early.

These phenomena may explain the individual rhythms of ageing for each of us, considering old age as a state of energy deficit. Most researchers have focused on the cell membrane in search of hypotheses to explain these observations. Researcher Sagan, in a personal paper (1990), listed some phenomena related to cell membrane functions including:

• changes in ion transport in the cell membrane, such as cellular Ca influx;

• reduction of cytotoxic lymphocyte cell surface receptors;

• diatomic mobility. In addition, there is some evidence of an effect on genetic transcription, and some researchers have claimed that there are some in vitro effects that could compromise the immune system, but the number of observations is small.

The significance of these observations could increase if there were other independent replicas of the various laboratories. The natural currents that come from the muscular activity of the heart or the neuro-transmitting activity of the brain are at an intensity of 10-100 mA / m, a much higher intensity than an intense current of 3 mA / m from the body's exposure to a field of 10 VK / sqm, common for any public person, in everyday life, at work.

A magnetic field can change the direction of motion of a charged particle, but it can never change its kinetic energy, so it would be surprising if an oscillating magnetic field had a greater effect on biological changes than an oscillating electric field. However, there is a possibility that electro-physiological processes in the body may be affected by exposure to weak magnetic or electric fields, but so far it is still difficult for us to prove that such influences can have effects on cellular transformations.

From a public health point of view, authors Ahlbom and Theriault, in the year 1999, concluded that the effects of the intense electromagnetic field could lead to an increase in cancer in children in the United States and Canada. However, it is considered that we do not have enough evidence at present for such quantification. Living matter is in constant motion, which is especially important for a magnetic field that generates electromotive forces in a moving conductor.

The orientation effects produced by external magnetic fields on paramagnetic molecules in the living matter can alter the rate of chemical reactions if it is accepted that Brownian agitation of molecules plays a role in the formation of chemical bonds. Setlow and Polland state that during a chemical reaction the rate of molecular rotation (rotational diffusion) increases by at least 10 times. If these molecules are paramagnetic, an external magnetic field can reduce rotational diffusion, reducing the permeability of affective bonds and delaying chemical reactions.

To completely stop a chemical reaction, after the author Valentizuzzi, 2002, a magnetic field with an intensity of 800,000 e (1Oe = 79.6 A / m) is required. The external magnetic field could also affect the chemical bonds already made, but in this case, it can be calculated that the interaction energy of the paramagnetic molecule with the external field of tens of thousands of Oe is many orders of magnitude smaller than the energy of the weakest. chemical bonds, H bond (4.5 Kcal/mol).

It is estimated that it is possible to inhibit the activity of enzymes due to changes in angles made by biochemical bonds and paramagnetic molecular stereochemical distortion. Magnetic fields would inhibit macromolecule biosynthesis through this mechanism, an effect observed by slowing down the rate of antibody production and the production of fibroblasts in the magnetic field.

It is also well known that the cell divides only when quantitative and qualitative into-cytoplasmic accumulations lead to a change in the cytoplasmic nucleus ratio by increasing the volume of the cytoplasm. Intense magnetic fields due to cumulative effects cause delays in cell growth, delays in regenerating damaged organs, and decreased tissue respiration. At the same time, the low-intensity cosmic-geomagnetic fields to which the body's cells adapt in amplitude and frequency determine beneficial effects:

• The exercise by the slightly intense magnetic fields of the specialized organs during the phylogenetic evolution in the conditions of the exposure to the terrestrial magnetic field leads to the orientation of the birds and mammals in space (diencephalic centres):

The effects on the genetic code regarding its stabilization in Blumenfeld's conception, regarding the pseudo-magnetism of nucleic acids, determine:

a) decrease in the incidence of carcinogenesis;

b) decrease in genetic anomalies;

c) inhibition of bacterial cultures during the stationary phase but especially in the logarithmic one;

d) delay in growth in biological age. The stabilizing effect of the magnetic field on the genetic code was confirmed by experiments with 42,000 Oe which led to the slowing down of ageing, and the preservation of the youth of the mice kept for 11 months in the magnetic field.

The direct action of the magnetic field on diencephalic structures has resulted in electrocardiographic and electroencephalographic changes. Intensity fields between 3000-4000 Oe delayed the development of transplanted malignancies (in plants). Although a well-differentiated magnetic analyzer has not yet been invented, these experiments demonstrate the sensitivity of cells or tissues to variations in the surrounding magnetic field. Experiments performed with the help of strong magnetic fields can

alter or mask this sensitivity and hence could come with the negative results often obtained by working methods with intense fields, [11].

3. Geomagnetism - the primary factor in the genesis of living matter

Our planet, including its living world, coexists in interrelationships with the cosmic environment with which it has a constant exchange of substance, energy, and information. The evolution of living matter is characterized by a permanent molecular chain reaction. In this evolutionary process, the magnetic head represented that "start" mechanism, so enigmatic and important for the processes in the body.

Everything alive on our planet depends on its magnetic field. The Earth's magnetic field can be likened to a huge umbrella that deflects cosmic radiation toward the earth. The natural radioactivity of the earth and cosmic rays amounts to 5 MeV, the electromagnetic potential required for the synthesis of adenine and nucleotides of nucleic acids. S.

Author Spiegelman in the year 2003, demonstrated that nucleic acids double "on their own" in their free environment with a protein coat and under the influence of electromagnetic radiation as the initial impulse for self-oscillations of biomolecules of cellular subcomponents that maintain internal order through enzymatic fluctuations. The human being during ontogenesis and phylogeny has been subjected to periodic variations of external factors and has evolved as a diurnal species.

The rotational motion of the Earth around its axis has determined over time the synchronization of several biological functions with a period of 24 hours (circadian rhythms), and the revolutionary movement of the Earth around the Sun and other planets around the Earth, through electromagnetic oscillations, printed certain biological characteristics and these were fixed in the fundamental structures of the cell (genome), thus becoming both in terms of functional rhythm (pace-maker) and in terms of the actions of environmental factors, with the mention that the environmental factors can influence the characteristic parameters of the biorhythms: periods, phases, etc., up to the level of a new functional adaptation.

Structural changes in nucleic acids and proteins based on certain legitimacies have facilitated the development of the theory of the existence of a probabilistic time "molecular clock of evolution" that marks the time of evolution. The frequency of molecular gene change is proportional to time

(Raicu, 1983).

It has been shown that the living organism, including the human body, manifests itself as a highly sensitive electromagnetic system that reacts to low-frequency geomagnetic variations. The oscillations of the geo-cosmic magnetic field range from 0.1 to 100 Hz. There is a relationship between electromagnetic fields caused by cosmic-geophysical pulsations and those emitted by the human brain (Antohi, 1984). This statement is based on the fact that cosmic geomagnetic phenomena are correlated and are similar to the frequency of electromagnetic oscillations emitted by the human brain in the range of 8-16 Hz and corresponding to the alpha rhythm.

The human body can be considered a biological oscillator subordinated to endogenous stimuli, respectively genetic signals (pacemaker) and environmental factors (Zeitheber, 1987). If the subject is suddenly taken out of its natural environment and relocated, the biological clock continues to operate for some time in the usual manner according to the schedule of the original place of origin until a new adaptation. The optimal level of adaptation and functioning of biological variations to the periodic phenomena of the internal or external environment results from the harmonious inhibition between endogenous oscillators and respectively the conditions of the environment.

The human body can be considered a universal biological oscillator because it is equipped and coded with various biological processes, from rhythms with a frequency of the order of milliseconds to rhythms with annual and multiannual periods. The triggering, maintenance, and directing of these cellular rhythms as well as their change in frequency and amplitude can be initiated and realized by the signals of the cosmos-geomagnetic and electromagnetic fields.

Against this background, in the absence of accidental factors, the death of living beings is due to its programming in the hereditary apparatus of the cell. With age, the rate of cell division decreases as a consequence of the loss of nuclear energy in cellular components, by the long disintegrations of γ radiation with the frequency and amplitude of each individual, **[Table 3].**

Table 3: *Biologic effect of quotidian magnetic field.*

Intensity, (Oe); 1 Oe-79.6 A/m	**Frequency (Hz)**
Geo-cosmic magnetic field necessary in assure DNA synthesis= 234 x 10^3	Geomagnetic field oscillations = 1-100 Hz
Magnetic field of earth = 0.5 Oe	Geomagnetic waves = 1-100 Hz
The maximum ground field in September =0.5 Oe	The maximum frequency of the geomagnetic field between 10 am and 6 pm = 100+100Hz
The minimum ground field in January = 0.05 Oe	Minimum frequency of the geomagnetic field between 4-15 hours =0.1-1 Hz
Magnetic field in malignant affection = 3-4 x10^3 Oe	Temporary magnetic storms = 5 x 10-6 Hz
A magnetic field with stabilizing effect on the genetic code = 4.2 x 10^3 Oe	Plasma magnetic waves = 0.001-1 x 10-6 Hz
$Magnetic\ field\ that\ can\ stop\ chemi$ $= 8x10-5\,Oe$	$The\ maximum\ froquoncy\ of\ c$ $= 4\,o'clock$
Magnetic field of magnetic bracelets = 2.5 x 10^2 Oe	Minimum frequency of cell mitosis and a maximum speed of DNA synthesis = 18 o'clock
Magnetic field of high voltage lines = 3 x 10-4 Oe	Frequency of the magnetic field of mitotic inhibition = 200 Hz
The magnetic field of the human brain = 1 x 10^{-3} Oe	Alpha, (α), frequency of the brain = 10 Hz
Horizontal geomagnetic components = 4 x 10-4 Oe	Frequencies needed for cosmic DNA synthesis = 1 x 10-6 Hz
Magnetic field in balneo physiological therapies = 6x 10………> 10 x 10 Oe	Frequency of magnetic field in balneary-physiotherapy recoveries = 50-100 Hz, (Direct and discontinuous current, alternating)

When the surrounding magnetism becomes lower, generally during the night, the G52 gene no longer inhibits the synthesis of the P-53 protein and degrades the division of the cell, which thus can no longer be stopped with the entry of the division protein, **[Figure 7]**.

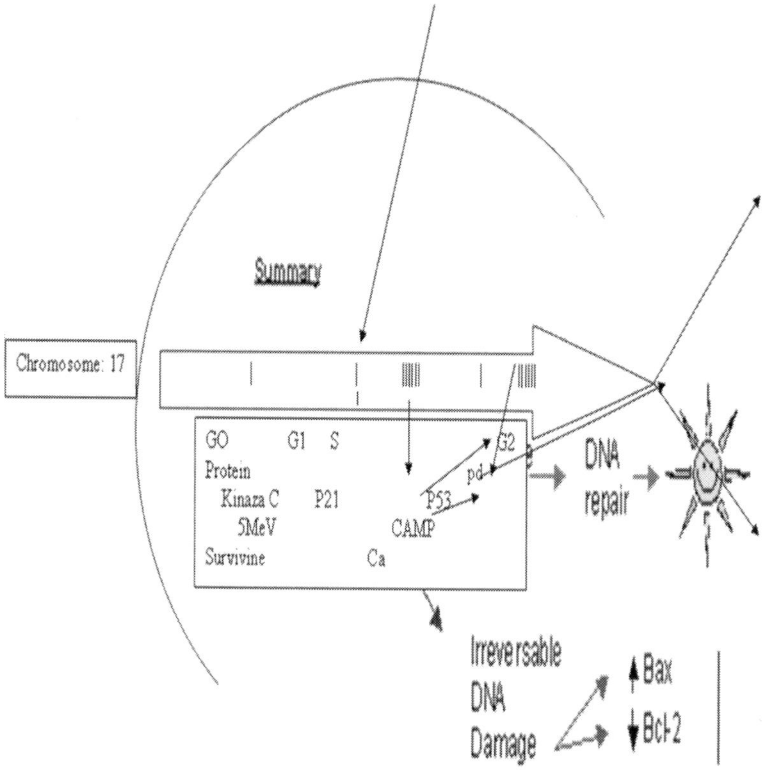

Fig5 Protein p21 is a cyclin-dependent kinase inhibitor that prevents cell cycle progression at G1. It is induced by wild-type p53 following DNA damage, and p21-null cells are deficient in DNA damage-induced, p53-mediated G1 arrest.

Figure 7. *The energy required for nuclear synthesis is 5 MeV and in this process, the protein kinase-C enzyme is of great importance which will trigger an intense phosphorylation activity of other proteins and enzymes involved in the key links of cellular metabolism.*

Explanatory note

• The cell has permanent metabolic oscillations under the influence of the geo-cosmic-magnetic field.

• The Earth, like the other planets in the Universe, has periodic magnetic pulsations with frequencies between 1-100 Hz. The planets bring magnetic waves of 1MHz to Earth, except for the Sun's magnetic storms, which can generate thousands of MHz waves for a short time.

• Cosmo-geomagnetic waves have maximum frequencies at 10.00 and 18.00 during the day, and the minimum frequencies are around 4.00 in the morning when in general the rhythm of cell divisions is maximum.

• The magnetic oscillator receptor sensor gene may be the G53 anti-oncogene, which by its product inhibits the P53 protein GD structural gene that will no longer synthesize the PD division protein in the post-synthetic G53 phase of the cell interface, and the cell remains in the mitotic waiting phase.

• When the surrounding magnetism becomes lower, generally during the night, the G52 gene no longer inhibits the synthesis of the PD protein and degrades the division of the cell, which thus can no longer be stopped with the entry of the division protein.

• The energy required for nuclear synthesis is 5 MeV and, in this process, the protein kinase-C enzyme is of great importance which will trigger an intense phosphorylation activity of other proteins and enzymes involved in the key links of cellular metabolism.

• In this way, the decrease in the reception of geo-cosmic magnetism by damaging the sensor gene is correlated with the initiation of anarchic multiplication by getting out of control of the structural gene GD producing the division protein.

• Increased magnetism in an intense electromagnetic field leads to anarchic cell proliferation by stimulating CAMP and ionic calcium, blocking cellular respiration, anaerobic environment favorable to neoplasia and enzymatic inhibition by the end product of normal pathways, with the initiation of other appropriate metabolic pathways and new stereochemical molecular structures modified by the magnetic field (ATPase 3 β).

• There is a gamma (γ) energy decay throughout the interface, so the new daughters will have a smaller isobaric nucleus with less nuclear energy than the original cell, and the longer the interface time, the more nuclear decay will be. intense after the cell has reached its maximum degree of maturation.

*The interaction between the magnetic flux and reflux from noon and midnight with living biological structures will be done through the esoteric double field that surrounds living matter. In this way, the high vibrational energy of negative space-temporality interferes with the genetic mechanisms that ensure the expression and continuity of life. The association of disaggregated astral energy with aggregate physical energy creates the nerve matter that is the cell, which gives the ability to feel pleasure and suffering.

As a result of thinking, of the higher dynamic cellular activity, the cells develop into cells and the bioenergy is distributed in three planes: physical, astral and mental. This magnetism maintains the circulation of etheric matter through the layer of ether that surrounds each cell. Life has more to it than people can imagine. However, man is constantly trying, through modern physical means, to enter the life of his higher self and to preserve in himself the glory of this higher self, continuing to live on this planet for as long as it exists.

Time is born of Universal Energy, the future passes over the existing humanity and from its past, a new humanity will be born, which will never meet the pre-existing humanity, so the "future" civilizations present the civilizations of the past on another planet, [12].

REFERENCES

1. Visnevschi A, Odiras S. Bioenergetic Lisosomale Proceses of Peroxid of Lypides and atioxidanr Sysrems of Soft Tissues on Beckground in Oxybar Medium . Ed. Ştiinţa Agricolă, nr. 2/2007. ISSN: 1857-0003.

2. Lehninger A. Biochimie vol I-II, Editura Tehnică, Bucureşti 1987-1992

3. V. Ranga; I. Teodorescu Exarcu. Anatomia şi fiziologia omului, Editura Medicală, Bucureşti 1970

4. Guide for Health Alimentation. Mariana Graur. Editura PERFORMANTICA, IAŞI 2006;ISBN: 973-730-240-4 ; 978-973-730-204-5.

5. Elena G, Bistriceanu A, Gorcea RV. Fiziologia normală şi patologică, Volumul 16,1970; 1: 190-332.

6. Jiang L, Mao XA. NMR evidence for Mg(II) binding to N1 of ATP. Spectrochim Acta A Mol Biomol Spectrosc. 2001 Jul;57(8):1711-6. doi: 10.1016/s1386-1425(01)00442-5.

7. Poenaru DV , MORFOPATOLOGIE GENERALĂ. Editura „Victor Babeş. © 2019. ISBN 978-606-786-150-1.

8. Cristescu D, Salavastru C, Voiculescu B. Manual de biologie. Bucure[ti: Corint Educa]ional, 2014. ISBN 978-606-8609-08

9. Mancas Malina. What are the difference? Benign and malignant tumors, link: https://www.cancercenter.com/discussions/blog/whats-the-difference-benign-and-malignant-tumors/Acceses in May 2021.

10. Novacu V. Electrodinamica; Capitolul VI, Cîmpul electromagnetic variabil. Editura didactică şi pedagogică, Bucureşti, 1966 p: 46-192

11. Manolachi E. Bioritmurile umane. Facultatea de Biologie si Pedologie. Chisinau 2017.

12. Dulcan DC. Inteligenta materiei. Cod: EIK973-757-222-6. Editura: EIKON. Bucuresti, 2020.

Made in the USA
Las Vegas, NV
22 March 2026

44054614R00129